IARC MONOGRAPHS
ON THE
EVALUATION OF THE CARCINOGENIC RISK
OF CHEMICALS TO MAN:

Sex hormones

Volume 6

This publication is the outcome of the meeting of the
IARC Working Group on the
Evaluation of the Carcinogenic Risk of Chemicals to Man,
Lyon, 4-11 February 1974

IARC WORKING GROUP ON THE EVALUATION OF THE CARCINOGENIC RISK OF CHEMICALS TO MAN: SEX HORMONES

Lyon, 4-11 February 1974

Members[1]

Dr H.A. Bern, Professor of Zoology, Research Endocrinologist in the Cancer Research Laboratory, University of California, Berkeley, California 94720, USA

Professor E. Boyland, London School of Hygiene and Tropical Medicine, Keppel Street, London WC1E 7HT, UK

Dr J.B. Brown, Department of Obstetrics and Gynaecology, University of Melbourne, Melbourne, Australia

Dr G.T. Bryan, Division of Clinical Oncology, University of Wisconsin Medical School, 1300 University Avenue, Madison, Wisconsin 53706, USA

Dr J.W. Jull, Cancer Research Center, University of British Columbia, Vancouver 8, British Columbia, Canada (Vice-Chairman)

Professor O. Muhlbock, The Netherlands Cancer Institute, Sarphatistraat 108, Amsterdam C, The Netherlands (Chairman)

Dr G. Rudali, Laboratoire de Génétique de la Fondation Curie, Institut du Radium, 26 rue d'Ulm, 75005 Paris, France

Dr P. Sartwell, Professor Emeritus of the Johns Hopkins School of Hygiene and Public Health, 615 North Wolfe Street, Baltimore, Maryland 21205, USA

Dr M. Vessey, Department of the Regius Professor of Medicine, University of Oxford, Radcliffe Infirmary, Oxford OX2 6HE, UK

Dr S.D. Vesselinovitch, Department of Radiology and Pathology, The University of Chicago, 950 East 59th Street, Chicago, Illinois 60637, USA

Dr B. Westerholm, Registration Division, Department of Drugs, National Board of Health and Welfare, 104-1 Stockholm 60, Sweden

---

[1] Unable to attend: Dr N.P. Napalkov, Petrov Research Institute of Oncology, Pesochny-2, Leningrad, USSR

Representative of the National Cancer Institute

Dr S. Siegel, Research Biologist, Carcinogen Bioassay and Program Resource Branch, Carcinogenesis DCCP, National Cancer Institute, National Institutes of Health, Bethesda, Maryland 20014, USA

Invited Guests

Dr P.S. Elias, Principal Medical Officer, Department of Health and Social Security, Alexander Fleming House, Elephant and Castle, London SE1 6BY, UK

Dr R. Kroes, Head of the Department of Oncology, Rijks Instituut voor de Volksgezondheid, Postbus 1, Bilthoven, The Netherlands

Dr K.E. McCaleb, Manager, Environmental Studies, Chemical Information Services, Stanford Research Institute, Menlo Park, California 94025, USA

Secretariat

    Dr C. Agthe, Unit of Chemical Carcinogenesis (Secretary)
    Dr H. Bartsch, Unit of Chemical Carcinogenesis
    Dr N. Day, Unit of Epidemiology and Biostatistics
    Dr J. Hilfrich, Unit of Chemical Carcinogenesis
    Dr E. Johannisson, Human Reproduction Unit, WHO
    Dr F.C. Lu, Food Additives Unit, WHO
    Dr E. de Maar, Drug Evaluation and Monitoring Unit, WHO
    Dr R. Montesano, Unit of Chemical Carcinogenesis
    Dr C.S. Muir, Chief, Unit of Epidemiology and Biostatistics
    Dr N. Muñoz, Unit of Biological Carcinogenesis
    Mrs C. Partensky, Unit of Chemical Carcinogenesis
    Dr L. Tomatis, Chief, Unit of Chemical Carcinogenesis
    Dr A.J. Tuyns, Unit of Epidemiology and Biostatistics
    Mr E.A. Walker, Unit of Environmental Carcinogens
    Mrs E. Ward, Editor
    Mr J.D. Wilbourn, Unit of Chemical Carcinogenesis

CONTENTS

	Page
BACKGROUND AND PURPOSE OF THE IARC PROGRAMME ON THE EVALUATION OF THE CARCINOGENIC RISK OF CHEMICALS TO MAN	7
SCOPE OF THE MONOGRAPHS	7
MECHANISM FOR PRODUCING THE MONOGRAPHS	8
Priority for the preparation of monographs	8
Data on which the evaluation is based	9
The Working Group	9
GENERAL REMARKS ON THE EVALUATION	9
Purity of the compounds tested	9
Terminology	9
Response to carcinogens	10
Qualitative aspects	10
Dose-response relationships	11
Animal data in relation to the evaluation of risk to man	11
Evidence of human carcinogenicity	11
EXPLANATORY NOTES ON THE MONOGRAPHS	12
GENERAL REMARKS ON THE SEX HORMONES	19
THE MONOGRAPHS	
Oestrogens:	
Diethylstilboestrol (Stilboestrol)	55
Ethinyloestradiol	77
Mestranol	87
Oestradiol-17β	99
Oestriol	117
Oestrone	123
Progestins:	
Progesterone	135

17-Hydroxyprogesterones:

    Chlormadinone acetate 149

    Medroxyprogesterone acetate 157

19-Nortestosterone derivatives:

    Dimethisterone 167

    Ethynodiol diacetate 173

    Norethisterone }
                           179
    Norethisterone acetate }

    Norethynodrel 191

    Norgestrel 201

Androgens:

    Testosterone 209

OESTROGENS AND PROGESTINS IN RELATION TO HUMAN CANCER 219

GENERAL CONCLUSIONS ON HORMONES 235

CUMULATIVE INDEX TO MONOGRAPHS 239

BACKGROUND AND PURPOSE OF THE IARC PROGRAMME ON THE
EVALUATION OF THE CARCINOGENIC RISK OF CHEMICALS TO MAN

The International Agency for Research on Cancer (IARC) initiated in 1971 a programme on the evaluation of the carcinogenic risk of chemicals to man. This programme was supported by a resolution of the Governing Council at its Ninth Session concerning the role of IARC in providing government authorities with expert, independent scientific opinion on environmental carcinogenesis. As one means to this end, the Governing Council recommended that IARC should continue to prepare monographs on the carcinogenic risk of individual chemicals to man.

In view of the importance of this programme and in order to expedite the production of monographs, the National Cancer Institute of the United States has provided IARC with additional funds for this purpose.

The aim of this programme is to arrive at and publish an objective evaluation of the available data through the deliberations of an international group of experts in chemical carcinogenesis, and to put into perspective the present state of knowledge with the final aim of evaluating the data in terms of possible human risk, as well as to indicate the need for research efforts to close the gaps in our knowledge.

SCOPE OF THE MONOGRAPHS

The monographs summarize the evidence for the carcinogenicity of individual chemicals. The data are compiled, reviewed and evaluated by a Working Group of experts. No recommendations are given concerning preventive measures of legislation, since these matters depend on risk-benefit evaluation, which seems best made by individual governments and /or international agencies such as WHO and ILO.

The first volume[1] covers a number of substances not belonging to a particular chemical group; the second[2], third[3], fourth[4] and fifth[5] volumes contain monogrpahs on: some inorganic and organometallic compounds; certain polycyclic aromatic hydrocarbons and heterocyclic compounds; some aromatic amines, hydrazine and related substances, N-nitroso compounds and miscellaneous alkylating agents; and some organochlorine pesticides, respectively. The present volume is devoted to some sex hormones.

As new data on chemicals for which monographs have already been written and new principles for evaluation become available, re-evaluations will be made at future meetings and revised monographs will be published as necessary. The monographs are being distributed to international and governmental agencies and will be available to industries and scientists dealing with these chemicals. They also form the basis of advice from IARC on carcinogenesis from these substances.

MECHANISM FOR PRODUCING THE MONOGRAPHS

As a first step, a list of chemicals for possible consideration by the Working Group is established. IARC then collects pertinent references regarding physico-chemical characteristics, production and use*, occurrence and analysis, and biological data** on these compounds. The material is summarized by an expert consultant or by an IARC staff member, who prepares the first draft monograph, which in some cases is sent to another expert for comments. The drafts are circulated to all members of the Working Group about one month before the meeting, during which further additions to and deletions from the data are agreed upon and a final version of comments and evaluation on each compound is adopted.

Priority for the Preparation of Monographs

Priority is given mainly to chemicals belonging to groups for which some experimental evidence of carcinogenicity exists and for which there is evidence of human exposure. However, neither human exposure nor potential carcinogenicity can be judged until all the relevant data have been collected

---

* Data provided by Chemical Information Services, Stanford Research Institute, Menlo Park, California, USA

** In the collection of original data reference was made to CBAC profile sheets, to the publications "Survey of Compounds which have been Tested for Carcinogenic Activity" [6,7,8,9,10,11] and to a bibliography provided by the Franklin Research Institute, USA

and examined in detail; and the inclusion of a particular compound in a monograph does not necessarily mean that the substance is considered to be carcinogenic. Equally, the fact that a substance has not yet been considered does not imply that it is without carcinogenic hazard.

Data on which the Evaluation is Based

With regard to the biological data, only published articles and papers already accepted for publication are reviewed. Every effort is made to cover the whole literature, but some studies may have been inadvertently overlooked. The monographs are not intended to be a full review of literature, and they contain only data considered relevant by the Committee. Research workers who are aware of important data (published or accepted for publication) which may influence the evaluation are invited to make them available to the Unit of Chemical Carcinogenesis of the International Agency for Research on Cancer, Lyon, France.

The Working Group

The members of the Working Group who participated in the consideration of particular substances are listed at the beginning of each publication. The members of the Working Group serve in their individual capacities as scientists, and not as representatives of their governments or of any organization with which they are affiliated.

GENERAL REMARKS ON THE EVALUATION

Purity of the Compounds Tested

In any evaluation of biological data with respect to a possible carcinogenic risk, particular attention must be paid to the purity of the chemicals tested and to their stability under conditions of storage or administration. Information on purity and stability is given, when available, in the monographs.

Terminology

The term "chemical carcinogenesis" in its widely accepted sense is used to indicate the induction or enhancement of neoplasia by chemicals. It is recognized that, in the strict etymological sense, this term means the induction of cancer. However, common usage has led to its employment to denote the induction of various types of neoplasms. The terms "tumourigen", "oncogen" and "blastomogen" have all been used synonymously with "carcinogen", although occasionally "tumourigen" has been used specifically to denote the induction of benign tumours.

Response to Carcinogens

For present purposes, in general, no distinction is made between the induction of tumours and the enhancement of tumour incidence, although it is noted that there may be fundamental differences in mechanisms that will eventually be elucidated.

The response in experimental animals to a carcinogen may take several forms:

(a) a significant increase in the incidence of one or more of the same types of neoplasms as found in control animals;
(b) the occurrence of types of neoplasms not observed in control animals;
(c) a decreased latent period as compared with control animals.

Qualitative Aspects

The qualitative nature of neoplasia has been much discussed. In many instances both benign and malignant tumours are induced by chemical carcinogens. There are so far few recorded instances in which only benign tumours are induced by chemicals that have been studied extensively. Their occurrence in experimental systems has been taken to indicate the possibility of an increased risk of malignant tumours also.

In experimental carcinogenesis, the type of cancer seen can be the same as that recorded in human studies (e.g., bladder cancer in man, monkeys, dogs and hamsters after administration of 2-naphthylamine). In other instances, however, a chemical can induce other types of neoplasms or neoplasms at different sites in various species (e.g., benzidine, which induces hepatic carcinoma in the rat, but bladder carcinoma in man).

Dose-Response Relationships

Dose-response studies are important in the evaluation of human and animal carcinogenesis. The confidence with which a carcinogenic effect can be established is strengthened by the observation of an increasing incidence of neoplasms with increasing exposure.

Animal Data in Relation to the Evaluation of Risk to Man

At the present time no attempt can be made to interpret the animal data directly in terms of human risk since no objective criteria are available to do so. The critical assessment of the validity of the animal data given in these monographs is intended to assist national and/or international authorities to make decisions concerning preventive measures or legislation. In this connection, attention is drawn to WHO recommendations in relation to food additives[12], drugs[13] and occupational carcinogens[14].

Evidence of Human Carcinogenicity

Evaluation of the carcinogenic risk to man of suspected environmental agents rests on purely observational studies. Such studies require sufficient variation in the levels of human exposure to allow a meaningful relationship between cancer incidence and exposure to a given chemical to be established. Difficulties in isolating the effects of individual agents arise, however, since populations are exposed to multiple carcinogens.

The initial suggestion of a relationship between an agent and disease often comes from case reports of patients who have had similar exposures. Variations and time trends in regional or national cancer incidence, or their correlation with regional or national exposure levels, may also provide valuable insights. Such observations by themselves, however, cannot in most circumstances be regarded as conclusive evidence of carcinogenicity. The most satisfactory epidemiological method is to compare the cancer risk (adjusted for age, sex and other confounding variables) among groups or cohorts, or among individuals exposed to various levels of the agent in question and among control groups not so exposed. Ideally this is accomplished directly, by following such groups forward in time (prospectively) to determine time relationships, dose-response relationships, and other aspects of cancer induction. Large cohorts and long observation periods are required to provide sufficient cases for a statistically valid comparison.

An alternative to prospective investigation is to assemble cohorts from past records and to evaluate their subsequent morbidity or mortality by means of medical histories and death certificates. Such occupational carcinogens as nickel, β-naphthylamine, asbestos and benzidine have been confirmed by this method. Another method is to compare the past exposures of a defined group of cancer cases with those of control samples from the hospital or general population. This does not provide an absolute measure of carcinogenic risk but can indicate the relative risks associated with different levels of exposure. The indirect means (e.g., interviews or tissue residues) used to measure exposures which may have commenced many years before can constitute a major source of error. Nevertheless such "case-control" studies can often isolate one factor from several suspected agents. The carcinogenic effect of this substance could then be confirmed by cohort studies.

EXPLANATORY NOTES ON THE MONOGRAPHS

In sections 1, 2 and 3 of each monograph, except for minor remarks, the data are recorded as given by the author, whereas the comments by the Working Group are given in section 4, headed "Comments on Data Reported and Evaluation".

Chemical and Physical Data (section 1)

The most important chemical synonyms and trade names are recorded in this section. The trade names are listed separately and include names of products containing mixtures.

Chemical and physical properties include data that might be relevant to carcinogenicity (for example, lipid solubility) and those that concern identification. Where applicable, data on solubility, volatility and stability are indicated. All chemical data in this section refer to the pure substances.

Production, Use, Occurrence and Analysis (section 2)

With regard to the data on use and occurrence of chemicals presented in the monographs, IARC has collaborated with the Stanford Research Institute, USA, with the support of the National Cancer Institute of the United States, in order to obtain production figures of chemicals and their patterns of use. These data more commonly refer to the United States and Western Europe than to other countries, solely as a result of the availability to the Working Group of more data from these countries than from others. It should not be implied that these nations are the sole sources or even the major sources of any individual chemical. In the case of drugs, mention of the therapeutic uses of such chemicals in this section does not necessarily represent presently accepted therapeutic indications, nor does it imply judgement as to their clinical efficacy.

In some countries, there are also legal restrictions on the conditions under which certain carcinogens, suspect chemicals and pesticides can be handled. Examples of these are given in section 2.2, when such information was available to the Working Group.

It is hoped that in future revisions of these monographs, more information on use and legislation can be made available to IARC from other countries.

Biological Data Relevant to the Evaluation of Carcinogenic Risk to Man (section 3)

As pointed out earlier in this introduction, the monographs are not intended to consider all studies reported in the literature. Although every effort was made to review the whole literature, some studies were purposely omitted (a) because of their inadequacy, as judged from previously described criteria[15,16,17,18] (e.g., too short a duration, too few animals, poor survival or too small a dose); (b) because they only confirmed findings which have already been fully described; or (c) because they were judged irrelevant for the purpose of the evaluation. However, in certain cases, reference is made to studies which did not meet established criteria of adequacy, particularly when this information was considered a useful supplement to other reports or when it may have been the only data available.

This does not, however, imply acceptance of the adequacy of experimental designs in these cases.

In general, the data recorded in this section are summarized as given by the author; however, certain shortcomings of reporting or of experimental design are also mentioned, and minor comments by the Working Group are given in brackets.

The essential comments by the Working Group are made in section 4, "Comments on Data Reported and Evaluation".

Carcinogenicity and related studies in animals (3.1)

Mention is usually made of all routes of administration by which the compound has been tested and of all aspects in which relevant tests have been carried out. In most cases the animal strains are given; general characteristics of mouse strains have been reported in a recent review[19]. Quantitative data are given in so far as they will enable the reader to realize the order of magnitude of the effective doses. In general, the doses are indicated as they appear in the original paper; sometimes conversions have been made for better comparison, and these are given in parentheses.

Other relevant biological data (3.2)

The reporting of metabolic data is restricted to studies showing the metabolic fate of the chemical in animals and man. Comparison of animal and human data is made when possible. Other metabolic information (e.g., absorption, storage and excretion) is given when the Working Group considered that it would enable the reader to have a better understanding of the fate of the compound in the body. When the carcinogenicity of known metabolites has been tested, this also is reported.

Data on toxicity are included occasionally, if considered relevant.

Observations in man (3.3)

Epidemiological studies are summarized. Clinical and other observations in man have been reviewed, when relevant.

Comments on Data Reported and Evaluation (section 4)

This section gives the critical view of the Working Group on the data reported. It should be read in conjunction with the data recorded and, in the case of the present volume, in conjunction with the section, "General Conclusions on Hormones".

Animal data (4.1)

The animal species mentioned are those in which the carcinogenicity of the substances was clearly demonstrated, irrespective of the route of administration. In the case of inadequate studies, when mentioned, comments to that effect are included. Routes of administration used in experimental animals that are similar to possible human exposure (ingestion, inhalation and skin exposure) are given particular mention. In most cases, tumour sites are also indicated. If the substance has produced tumours on pre-natal exposure or in single-dose experiments, this is also indicated.

Human data (4.2)

In some cases, a brief statement is made on the possible exposure of man. The significance of epidemiological studies and case reports is discussed, and the data are interpreted in terms of possible human risk.

References

1. IARC (1972) *IARC Monographs on the Evaluation of Carcinogenic Risk of Chemicals to Man, 1*, Lyon

2. IARC (1973) *IARC Monographs on the Evaluation of Carcinogenic Risk of Chemicals to Man, 2, Some Inorganic and Organometallic Compounds*, Lyon

3. IARC (1973) *IARC Monographs on the Evaluation of Carcinogenic Risk of Chemicals to Man, 3, Certain Polycyclic Aromatic Hydrocarbons and Heterocyclic Compounds*, Lyon

4. IARC (1974) *IARC Monographs on the Evaluation of Carcinogenic Risk of Chemicals to Man, 4, Some Aromatic Amines, Hydrazine and Related Substances, N-nitroso Compounds and Miscellaneous Alkylating Agents*, Lyon

5. IARC (1974) *IARC Monographs on the Evaluation of Carcinogenic Risk of Chemicals to Man, 5, Some Organochlorine Pesticides*, Lyon

6. Hartwell, J.L. (1951) *Survey of compounds which have been tested for carcinogenic activity*, Washington DC, US Government Printing Office (Public Health Service Publication No. 149)

7. Shubik, P. & Hartwell, J.L. (1957) *Survey of compounds which have been tested for carcinogenic activity*, Washington DC, US Government Printing Office (Public Health Service Publication No. 149: Supplement 1)

8. Shubik, P. & Hartwell, J.L. (1969) *Survey of compounds which have been tested for carcinogenic activity*, Washington DC, US Government Printing Office (Public Health Service Publication No. 149: Supplement 2)

9. Carcinogenesis Program National Cancer Institute (1973) *Survey of compounds which have been tested for carcinogenic activity*, Washington DC, US Government Printing Office (Public Health Service Publication No. 149: 1961-1967)

10. Thompson, J.I. & Co. (1971) *Survey of compounds which have been tested for carcinogenic activity*, Washington DC, US Government Printing Office (Public Health Service Publication No. 149: 1968-1969)

11. Carcinogenesis Program National Cancer Institute (1974) *Survey of compounds which have been tested for carcinogenic activity*, Washington DC, US Government Printing Office (Public Health Service Publication No. 149: 1970-1971) (in press)

12. WHO (1961) Fifth Report of the Joint FAO/WHO Expert Committee on Food Additives. Evaluation of carcinogenic hazard of food additives. Wld Hlth Org. techn. Rep. Ser., No. 220, pp. 5, 18, 19

13. WHO (1969) Report of a WHO Scientific Group. Principles for the testing and evaluation of drugs for carcinogenicity. Wld Hlth Org. techn. Rep. Ser., No. 426, pp. 19, 21, 22

14. WHO (1964) Report of a WHO Expert Committee. Prevention of cancer. Wld Hlth Org. techn. Rep. Ser., No. 276, pp. 29, 30

15. WHO (1958) Second Report of the Joint FAO/WHO Expert Committee on Food Additives. Procedures for the testing of intentional food additives to establish their safety for use. Wld Hlth Org. techn. Rep. Ser., No. 144

16. WHO (1961) Fifth Report of the Joint FAO/WHO Expert Committee on Food Additives. Evaluation of carcinogenic hazard of food additives. Wld Hlth Org. techn. Rep. Ser., No. 220

17. WHO (1967) Scientific Group. Procedures for investigating intentional and unintentional food additives. Wld Hlth Org. techn. Rep. Ser., No. 348

18. UICC (1969) Carcinogenicity testing. UICC techn. Rep. Ser., Vol. 2

19. Committee on Standardized Genetic Nomenclature for Mice (1972) Standardized nomenclature for inbred strains of mice. Fifth listing. Cancer Res., 32, 1609-1646

GENERAL REMARKS ON THE SEX HORMONES

Introduction

The compounds considered in this section are listed in Table I. With the exception of diethylstilboestrol, they are steroid derivatives. They have all been used in some form of therapy in humans, and those marked with an asterisk have found widespread use as oral hormonal contraceptive agents.

In considering their carcinogenic activity, it is necessary to relate their pathogenic activities to their varying physiological properties. The naturally occurring oestrogens, oestradiol and oestrone, the natural androgen, testosterone, and the natural progestin, progesterone, are present in all vertebrate species as secretions of the ovary, testis and adrenal gland and are products of the mammalian placenta. As such, they form part of the total endocrine environment, the inter-relationships and control of which are complex. For background information the reader may consult Turner & Bagnara (1971), and for more detailed accounts of the steroid hormones the works of Applezweig (1962,1964) and Briggs & Brotherton (1970) are comprehensive.

Essentially the compounds considered are oestrogens, androgens or progestins (progestogens), and the general activities of these three classes of compounds are outlined below in relation to growth, differentiation and development. It is important to realize that classification of hormones with regard to these types of biological activity cannot be rigid since it is based on a number of physiological properties which individual compounds may possess to varying degrees. In addition, activity in different systems often varies according to the route of administration, the vehicle used and the species, sex and strain of test animals.

Effects of oestrogens

Oestrogens are responsible, together with other hormones, for the maintenance of the female sex organs and for the regulation of the menstrual cycle in primates and of the oestrus cycle in other mammals.

TABLE I

LIST OF COMPOUNDS REVIEWED

Compound	CAS[†] No.	CAS[†] preferred nomenclature
Oestrogens		
Diethylstilboestrol	56531	4,4'-(1,2-Diethyl-1,2-ethenediyl)bis-phenol
Ethinyloestradiol*	57636	(17α)-19-Norpregna-1,3,5(10)-trien-20-yne-3,17-diol
Mestranol*	72333	3-Methoxy-(17α)-19-norpregna-1,3,5(10)-trien-20-yn-17-ol
Oestradiol-17β	50282	(17β)-Oestra-1,3,5(10)-triene-3,17-diol
Oestriol	50271	(16α,17β)-Oestra-1,3,5(10)-triene-3,16,17-triol
Oestrone	53167	3-Hydroxy-oestra-1,3,5(10)-trien-17-one
Progestins		
Chlormadinone acetate*	302227	17-(Acetyloxy)-6-chloro-pregna-4,6-diene-3,20-dione
Dimethisterone*	79641	17-Hydroxy-6-methyl-17-(1-propynyl)-(6α,17β)androst-4-en-3-one
Ethynodiol diacetate*	297767	(3β,17α)-19-Norpregn-4-en-20-yne-3,17-diol diacetate
Medroxyprogesterone acetate*	71589	17-(Acetyloxy)-6-methyl-(6α)-pregn-4-ene-3,20-dione
Norethisterone*	68224	17-Hydroxy-(17α)-19-norpregn-4-en-20-yn-3-one
Norethisterone acetate*	51989	17-Hydroxy-(17α)-19-norpregn-4-en-20-yn-3-one acetate
Norethynodrel*	68235	17-Hydroxy-(17α)-19-norpregn-5(10)-en-20-yn-3-one
Norgestrel*	797637	13-Ethyl-17-hydroxy(17α)-18,19-dinorpregn-4-en-20-yn-3-one
Progesterone	57830	Pregn-4-ene-3,20-dione
Androgens		
Testosterone	58220	17-Hydroxy-(17β)-androst-4-en-3-one

* Used in oestrogen-progestin oral contraceptive preparations
† Chemical Abstracts Service

Oestrogens produce marked proliferative effects in all tissues derived from the Mullerian duct system. In the uterus, oestrogens initially induce fluid retention and stimulation of epithelial multiplication. The endometrium becomes thickened and highly vascularized. In menstruating species the glands elongate and glycogen is formed in the gland cells, but they do not secrete. The secretion of cervical mucous is stimulated, and in the absence of progestin this constitutes a most sensitive indicator of oestrogenic activity. The multiplication of vaginal epithelial cells is stimulated, the infiltration of leucocytes is inhibited and there is keratinization in rodents.

In the secondary sex tissues, oestrogens are responsible for proliferation of the ducts in the breast and for an increase in the size and pigmentation of the nipples. In the human female, oestrogens are responsible for the typical distribution of fat in the breast and hips and for the regulation of characteristic hair growth.

Oestrogens have a wide variety of effects on other organs, as shown by studies with the synthetic oestrogens used in oral contraceptives. For example, oestrogens influence the cardiovascular system, and they increase the incidence of thrombosis. They affect liver function in many ways. They also affect carbohydrate and mineral metabolism, serum lipids and proteins and influence the factors involved in blood coagulation. Comprehensive reviews of this complex topic are available (WHO, 1971, 1973).

Oestrogens have marked effects on the hypothalamus, which in turn regulates the release of follicle-stimulating hormone (FSH) and luteinizing hormone (LH) by the pituitary. Low levels may be stimulatory and high levels inhibitory. Under continuous dosage, inhibiting gonadotrophin secretion, the ovaries become smaller and non-functioning; however, this effect is usually immediately reversed upon removal of the inhibition. Oestrogens also influence the release of prolactin, which may have effects on a number of tissues.

Biological assays for oestrogens are based either on the induction of vaginal keratinization or on the increase in uterine weight induced in immature or ovariectomized rats or mice. One rat unit represents approximately 0.1 µg oestradiol, but this depends on the assay.

Effects of progestins

Progesterone is the only important natural progestin, but many synthetic steroids have similar biological properties. The normal role of progesterone is to prepare the uterus for implantation and to maintain pregnancy. To achieve this normal response, prior stimulation with oestrogen is essential. The action of progesterone on the oestrogen-primed uterus is to induce further development of the endometrial glands and the secretion of glycogen into the uterine cavity; further action leads to the decidual changes. The maintenance of pregnancy is dependent on continuing progesterone production in sufficient amounts.

Progesterone acts as a potent anti-oestrogen on endocervical secretion and rapidly inhibits both the quantity and quality of the fertile-type mucus induced at the oestrogen peak at mid-cycle. Progesterone causes proliferation of acini in the oestrogen-stimulated ducts of the breast; it may also inhibit prolactin release from the pituitary and thus inhibit lactation. Raised progestin levels inhibit the release of LH at mid-cycle, and higher levels inhibit FSH production. Progestins acting without prior oestrogen priming have effects on the uterine endometrium which are obviously different from normal.

Bioassays for progestins are less satisfactory than those for the other hormones. They are conducted on oestrogen-primed animals, and the end-point may be either glandular endometrial proliferation, deciduoma formation or the maintenance of pregnancy.

Effects of androgens

Testosterone is the most potent natural androgen, although androgenic activity is present in varying degrees in many of its derivatives. Androgens are necessary for the maintenance of germinal tissue in the testis and for the differentiation and growth of the secondary sex organs in the male. Vestigial remnants of the male accessory tissues in the female are stimulated by androgens, and it is probable that low levels of androgenic activity form an essential component of the normal female hormone environment. Development of the prostate and seminal vesicles and of their secretion is stimulated by androgens. Secretion by the sebaceous glands is also increased, and pigmentation of the skin is stimulated. The characteristic distribution and growth of hair in the male are determined by androgenic activity.

Androgens have a marked anabolic effect, with increased protein synthesis, particularly in muscle and bone, resulting in an increased rate of body growth. There is retention of nitrogen, phosphorous and potassium and an increased use of body fat for protein synthesis.

In females androgens have activities comparable to those of the progestins in the breast, uterus and vagina. In addition, they stimulate hypertrophy of the clitoris.

Biological activities of steroid hormone preparations

The compounds listed in Table I have varying degrees of oestrogenic, androgenic or progestational activity. The degrees of activity depend on the route of administration and on the animal used. Furthermore, metabolites of the administered compounds may themselves have important physiological effects, depending on the animal used. Because of these factors, it is practically impossible to calculate accurate relative potencies in the human from animal data. Usually a better guide is to consider the doses of hormones used therapeutically, for example, the amounts required in oral contraception to inhibit ovulation. Nevertheless, for interest, some of the reported data relating potencies of the various hormone preparations are given in Tables II, III and IV.

The relative potencies of the oestrogenic substances listed in Table II were based on augmentation of uterine weight in ovariectomized, immature rats and on vaginal keratinization. The progestin activities listed in Table III were based on the following four, different types of assay:

1. The compound was injected subcutaneously in oestrogen-primed, immature rabbits, the end-point being the degree of glandular proliferation in the uterus compared to that induced by progesterone (Clauberg, 1930; McPhail, 1935).

2. As for 1., except that the compound was administered orally and the standard of reference was ethisterone, which has approximately 15 times the activity of progesterone.

TABLE II

RELATIVE OESTROGENIC POTENCIES

(based on Briggs & Brotherton, 1970)

	Method	
	Uterine weight	Vaginal keratinization
Oestradiol-17β	8	10
Oestrone	9	1
Oestriol	2	0.1
Ethinyloestradiol	10	10
Mestranol*	-	-
Diethylstilboestrol	14	-

* Probably comparable with ethinyloestradiol

TABLE III

PROGESTIN ACTIVITY

	Method[#]			
	1	2	3	4
Progesterone	1		1	1
Chlormadinone acetate	50*	175		
Medroxyprogesterone acetate	50-60	10-15	25	30-45
Norethisterone	0.5	5	<1	0.1
Norethynodrel	0.25	1.5	0	1.5[†]
Norgestrel		5		
Dimethisterone		3		
Ethynodiol diacetate				

* from Briggs & Brotherton (1970)

[†] oral dosage compared to ethisterone

[#] for details of the methods used see pp. 23, 27

All other date from Applezweig 1962, or 1964

TABLE IV

RELATIVE BIOLOGICAL EFFECTS OF SOME PROGESTINS

(from Nelson, 1973)

Compound	Oestro-genic	Anti-oestrogenic	Andro-genic	Progesta-tional
Norethynodrel	++	-	-	±
Norethisterone	-	+	+	+
Norethisterone acetate	-	++	+	+
Ethynodiol diacetate	+	++	+	++
Norgestrel	-	+++	+	++++

3. The compound was introduced surgically directly into the uterine lumen of oestrogen-primed, immature rabbits and was retained by sutures. The end-point was the degree of glandular proliferation induced compared to that induced by progesterone (McGinty et al., 1939).

4. The elevation of levels of uterine carbonic anhydrase produced by the injected compound was compared to that produced by progesterone (Elton, 1959).

Nelson (1973) assessed the relative biological activities of some of the more common progestins, and these are reproduced in Table IV. It should be emphasized again that certain biological functions may be due not to the compound tested but to its metabolism to other biologically active compounds, or to the presence of impurities in the specimen tested. Thus, Brazeau et al. (1973) have shown that the repeated crystallization of commercial norethynodrel induces more rapid clotting of blood in rats.

The role of hormones in tumour induction

Steroid hormones and those synthetic steroidal or non-steroidal compounds with hormonal activity interact closely with the secretions of the anterior pituitary and other endocrine secretions to modify the growth and secretory activity of many tissues. In the absence of the requisite hormonal environment and, thus, with incomplete or absent proliferation, other carcinogenic agents may be unable to act. It is, therefore, difficult in experimental tumour induction to dissociate the effects of the hormones themselves from the effects of other agents, such as chemicals, viruses or radiation, to which the test animals may be exposed.

It should be borne in mind that not only may hormones be synergistic for the action of other carcinogens, but, alternatively, that other cancer-inducing agents may act by distributing the hormonal balance, so that hormonal factors are the effective cause of neoplasia. An example of this type of action is the effect of DMBA (7,12-dimethylbenz(a)anthracene) on the mouse ovary, where it probably acts to eliminate the ova, thus producing a state of hyperstimulation by the pituitary gonadotrophins; the resulting granulosa-cell tumours are thus a consequence of the excessive gonadotrophin stimulation (see review by Jull, 1973).

In assessing the effects of hormones on the induction of tumours of the breast and of the haemopoietic system in mice, the interaction of viral factors has been shown to be of decisive importance. In the case of mammary tumourigenesis, the presence of a milk-borne virus (the mammary tumour virus, or MTV) has been established for many years, but there is good reason to suppose that at least one other viral factor, the nodule-inducing virus (or NIV), may also play a vital role. The NIV is not transmitted via the mother's milk, and therefore NIV-free strains of mice cannot be obtained by foster-nursing (see review by Nandi, 1965).

Hormones, including the steroids, may affect the action of chemical carcinogens by modifying their metabolism. The production of proximate carcinogenic metabolites might possibly be reduced or eliminated (Weisburger, 1968). Similar effects of hormonal treatment on the activity of environmental carcinogens must therefore be considered before attributing the carcinogenic activity of administered hormones to a direct action by the compounds themselves.

Hormones may precipitate neoplasia:

(a) by a direct carcinogenic action;

(b) by stimulating the production of other hormonal factors which, in excess, cause cancer;

(c) by acting synergistically to promote growth in tissues affected by a physical, chemical or viral carcinogen;

(d) by modifying the metabolism of chemical agents so that they become active carcinogens; or

(e) by modifying immune responses.

Relative activities of steroid hormones in various animal species

The differences which occur in the basic endocrine relationships in a range of laboratory animal species as compared to those in man have been discussed at length by Neumann & Elger (1972). Differences among species in the rates of absorption, metabolism and excretion of such compounds also exist (Kolb, 1972), resulting in unpredictable variations in the duration and level of exposure to the same drug administered at the same dose:weight ratio by the same route necessary to produce similar results in different species. Comparative studies of the metabolism of steroid hormones in man and animals have been reported by Breuer (1972), introducing a further parameter affecting the biological potency of steroids in different species.

The significance of mammary nodules in the female dog

The majority of studies on mammary tumour induction in dogs has been made in female beagles. Finkel & Berliner (1973) have outlined the historical development of the requirements of this system in drug testing, and they give tables listing the incidences of palpable nodules in the breasts of dogs given dosages of synthetic progestins at 1, 10 or 25 times the human dose, over periods of one to five years. Untreated dogs were examined over the same period and in a similar manner.

In general, the results of their studies up to February 1973 indicate that the oestrogens, mestranol and ethinyloestradiol, have had no nodule-inducing potential. The 19-nortestosterone derivatives, norethisterone, norethynodrel and norgestrel, have also shown no effect on the numbers of nodules occurring. Contrarily, a number of progesterone-related synthetic progestins have had marked tumourigenic potential in the dog breast. Chlormadinone acetate and megestrel acetate induced nodules beginning in the second and third year of administration, and some of these were revealed by biopsy to be benign or malignant tumours. Intramuscular injection of medroxyprogesterone acetate produced malignant nodules with metastases in an unspecified number of cases. Chloroethynyl norgestrel and anagestone acetate also had tumourigenic activity.

Nelson et al. (1973) have described in detail the occurrence of palpable nodules following progestin treatment and have evaluated 60 of these lesions by detailed histological study. Thirty-nine were classified as nodular hyperplasia, nine as benign, mixed, mammary tumours and only one as an adenocarcinoma. Their morphological descriptions emphasize the frequency of myoepithelial proliferation. They point out that evaluation of tumourigenic activity, on a count of mammary nodules only, can be grossly misleading.

It has been stated (Vallance & Capel-Edwards, 1971) that progesterone also induces mammary hyperplasia when given over a period of 74 weeks at high dosages. Later studies have not been reported.

In evaluating the utility of mammary-nodule or tumour induction in female dogs a number of moderating factors should be borne in mind. The well-known susceptibility of dogs to benign and malignant mammary tumours has been documented by Andersen (1965) and by Cotchin (1962). It may be related to the fact that dogs have only one or two periods of oestrus per year and that these are commonly followed by pseudopregnancy lasting for several months. A protracted period of endogenous progesterone secretion may thus provide the basis for the common occurrence of mammary hyperplastic lesions.

In the case of chlormadinone acetate, it has been shown (Dorfman, 1972) that the progestational activity of this compound in beagles is much greater than is that of norethisterone. Using several parameters of utero-trophic potency, he concluded that chlormadinone acetate was 30 times more potent as a progestin in dogs than was norethisterone; conversely, in women, the relative progestational activity of chlormadinone acetate: norethisterone was stated to be only 5:1.

It may be concluded that the breast tissue of dogs is unusually susceptible to tumour induction by progestins. Tumour-inducing properties of a steroid in this system thus provide an extremely sensitive index of progesterone-like activity which is not necessarily related to its carcinogenic hazard in other species.

Physiological production of sex hormones in the human

The normal menstrual cycle

A characteristic pattern of interdependent fluctuating hormone levels is found during the fertile ovarian cycle. This is illustrated in Figure 1. The cycle commences with a small rise in FSH production, which reaches 10 to 30% above threshold level. This causes follicles within the ovary to develop and to secrete increasing amounts of oestrogen, which then depress the FSH production below the threshold level. The oestrogen secretion

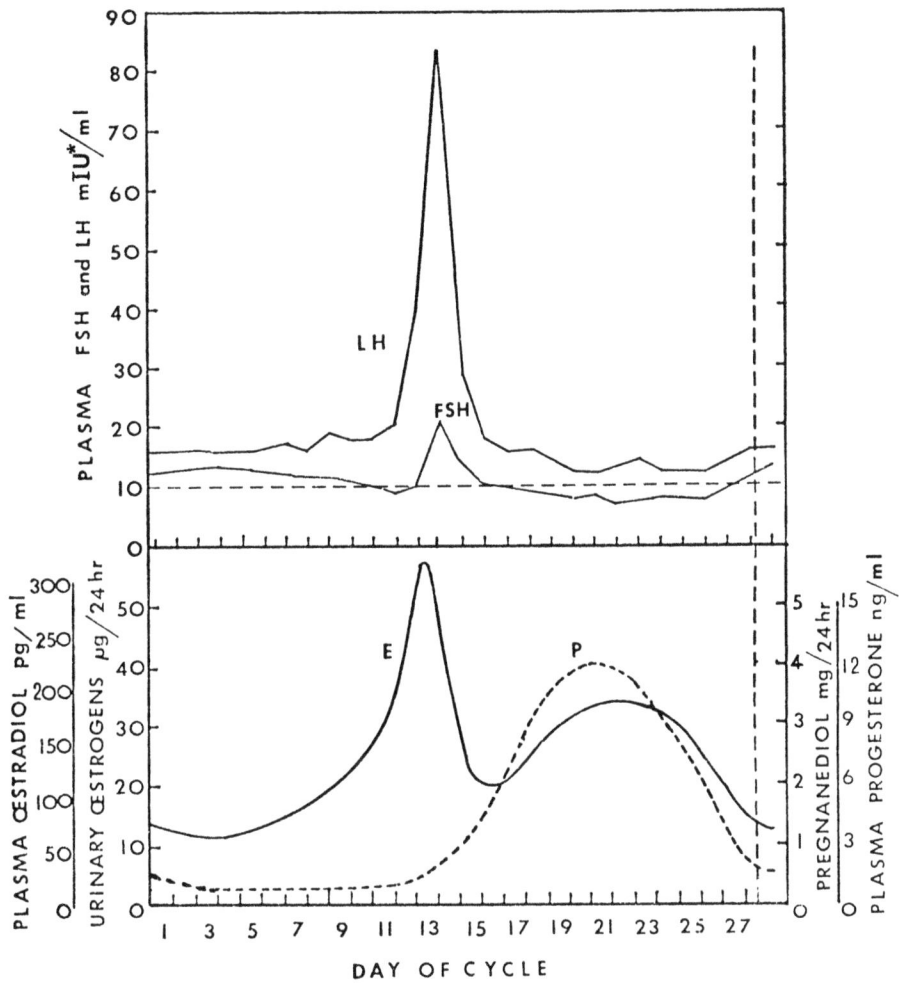

Figure 1. The natural sequence of FSH, LH, oestradiol (E) and progesterone (P) during the ovulatory cycle in women expressed as plasma concentrations. Urine concentrations of the steroid metabolites are also given.

Horizontal broken line = threshold level of FSH below which no follicular development occurs

Vertical broken line = onset of menstruation

Data of FSH and LH are from Ross et al. (1970), and the plasma and urine concentrations are means from the literature.

* Milli International Units

reaches a peak and then falls. During this time the dominant follicle is acquiring increasing sensitivity to LH. The elevated oestrogen levels act on the hypothalamus to produce LH-releasing factor, which triggers the massive release of LH which induces ovulation. This LH peak is accompanied by a smaller peak in FSH. After ovulation the developing corpus luteum produces increasing amounts of oestrogen and progesterone, which rise to a maximum and then fall before the onset of menstruation.

The concentrations of oestradiol, oestrone and progesterone in the plasma and of their metabolites in the urine at various stages of the cycle are shown in Table V, the values being the means of reported figures. The daily production rates, which are more closely related to physiological action, are also shown and are calculated from the data of Baird et al. (1969).

Most of the oestradiol in peripheral plasma (94%) is derived from secreted oestradiol, and the remainder is derived by conversion from oestrone. The oestrone in peripheral plasma is derived partly (70%) from secreted oestrone, partly (23%) by conversion from oestradiol and partly (7%) by conversion from androstenedione (Baird et al., 1969). Oestradiol is the major (90%) oestrogen secreted by the ovaries with concentrations in ovarian vein blood 10 to 20 times those in peripheral blood. Practically no progesterone is secreted by the ovaries during the follicular phase, but during the luteal phase the concentrations of progesterone in ovarian vein blood are 10 to 20 times those in peripheral blood (Lloyd et al., 1971). Secretion of oestradiol and progesterone by the ovaries occurs episodically, and definite fluctuations in plasma levels occur over short periods of time (Korenman & Sherman, 1973; West et al., 1973).

The total production of oestradiol during a 28-day cycle amounts to 5.0 mg, of which 0.9 mg is produced during the first 9 days, 1.6 mg are produced during the 6 days of the mid-cycle peak and 2.5 mg are produced during the 13 days of the luteal phase. The total ovarian production of progesterone during the luteal phase amounts to 230 mg. These calculations are based on the population means shown in Figure 1. For corresponding days of the cycle, the steroid values found in a female population vary over a

TABLE V

PLASMA CONCENTRATIONS AND PRODUCTION RATES (BPR) OF OESTRADIOL-17β, OESTRONE, PROGESTERONE AND TESTOSTERONE AND URINE EXCRETIONS OF 'TOTAL' OESTROGENS AND PREGNANEDIOL IN WOMEN AND MEN

	OESTRADIOL-17β		OESTRONE		PROGESTERONE		TESTOSTERONE		'TOTAL' URINE	
	Plasma pg/ml	BPR μg/24hr	Plasma pg/ml	BPR μg/24hr	Plasma ng/ml	BPR mg/24hr	Plasma ng/100ml	BPR mg/24hr	Oestrogens μg/24 hr	Pregnanediol mg/24 hr
Women										
Early follicular phase	65	85	60	130	0.6	1.2	40	0.3	15	0.4
Mid-cycle E peak	260	340	100	220					60	0.7
Luteal maximum	150	200	100	220	13	26			45	4.0
Post-menopause	5	5	17	30	0.3	0.6			7	0.2
Late Pregnancy	18,000	80,000*	6,000	80,000*	100	200			30,000	45
Men	20	50	30	55	0.4	0.8	660	6.6	15	0.5

* Total oestriol, oestrone and oestradiol-17β

Values for plasma concentrations are means from the literature, and the BPR's were calculated from the data of Baird et al. (1969).

Values for urine from Brown et al. (1968) and from Barrett & Brown (1970)

3- to 4-fold range, so that the upper limits of normal levels can be calculated approximately by multiplying the mean values by 2 and the lower limits by dividing them by 2.

In normal women, the mean plasma testosterone level is 40 ng per 100 ml, and the daily production rate is 0.3 mg. Only 27% of this is derived from secreted testosterone, the remainder being derived by conversion from other androgens (Baird et al., 1969). The secreted testosterone is derived in part from the ovaries, the concentration in ovarian vein blood being approximately 4 times that in peripheral blood (West et al., 1973).

Anovulatory menstrual cycles

Anovulatory cycles are characterized by the absence of the normal increases in progesterone production during the luteal phase. Two main patterns of oestrogen production have been described (Brown & Matthew, 1962). One shows constantly elevated oestrogen values and bleeding, usually irregularly, as a break-through phenomenon. The other shows a single peak of oestrogen production with maximum values which sometimes exceed those of the normal cycle, and oestrogen withdrawal bleeding occurs as the values fall after the peak. There are many variants of this pattern, however: a small transient increase in progesterone production may sometimes be observed after the oestrogen peak; but all gradations occur, from this small increase, through an inadequate luteal phase to the full pattern of the ovulatory cycle. In the intermediate patterns it may be difficult to decide whether ovulation has occurred or not. The gonadotrophin patterns are variable: the early rise in FSH may be delayed or absent, or the mid-cycle peaks of LH and FSH may be reduced or absent (Faiman & Ryan, 1967). The total oestrogen production throughout anovulatory cycles does not exceed that of the upper range of the ovulatory cycle, even in those with temporary high values; thus the condition is not associated with excessive oestrogen production but with absent progesterone production.

Post-menopausal women, ovariectomized women and women with prolonged amenorrhea

These conditions are characterized by absence of ovarian activity and by very low production of oestrogens and progesterone (Table V). Oestrone accounts for 85% of the free plasma oestrogens and is derived largely by peripheral conversion from androstenedione; the remainder probably arises from direct secretion of oestrone by the adrenals (Longcope, 1971).

Men

The relevant data for men are shown in Table V. The high plasma testosterone values are derived almost entirely from the secretion of testosterone by the testes (Baird et al., 1969). Much of the production of oestradiol and oestrone is accounted for by peripheral conversion of testosterone from the testes and of androstenedione from the adrenals. However, oestradiol is secreted directly by the testes, and this accounts for approximately 25% of the total oestradiol produced (Kelch et al., 1972; Longcope et al., 1972).

Children

Oestrogens levels in young children are below the sensitivity of current methods of measurement, and no reliable data are available on plasma or urinary levels or on production rates. Oestrogen output in girls rises steadily throughout puberty, which is initiated by increased gonadotrophin excretion, especially of FSH (Jenner et al., 1972). The early cycles are anovulatory, but ovulatory cycles become more common and reach the frequency of adult fertile women by the age of 18 years.

Pregnant women

Pregnancy is characterized by the production of relatively enormous amounts of oestrogens and progesterone. Thus, at term, the total daily productions of oestrogens and progesterone are of the order of 100 and 200 mg, respectively (Brown, 1957; Lin et al., 1972). In very early pregnancy, the luteal phase levels of oestrogens and progesterone are maintained. However, the growing placenta produces increasing amounts of these steroids and also of oestriol and by the 6th week becomes the major site of hormone production. The proportion of oestriol to total oestrogens increases as pregnancy advances, and at term oestriol accounts for 70% of the total production (Brown, 1957). Placental oestradiol and oestrone are derived by aromatization of dehydroepiandrosterone secreted by the foetal adrenals, and the oestriol is produced from the same compound after being 16-hydroxylated by the foetal liver (the 'feto-placental unit' (Diczfalusy, 1969)). The mean plasma concentrations of unconjugated oestradiol, oestrone and oestriol in the maternal circulation at term are 18, 6 and 12 ng per ml, respectively, and 99, 97 and 82% of these are bound to protein. Concentrations of the unbound unconjugated oestrogens are 3 to 6 times higher in the foetal than in the maternal circulation, indicating that the foetus is exposed to high plasma concentrations of these oestrogens (Tulchinsky, 1973).

Pregnancy is also characterized by the production by the placenta of large amounts of human chorionic gonadotrophin (HCG) and of human placental lactogen. The production of HCG can be detected as early as 10 days after ovulation (Thomas et al., 1973).

Pharmacology of the synthetic oestrogens and progestins

The synthetic oestrogens and progestins considered here are listed in Table I. The doses commonly used in gynaecological treatment or in combinations for hormonal contraception are listed in Table VI. It can be assumed that the doses listed are near the minimum required for suppression of ovulation and therefore have the same order of biological activity as the maximum levels found during the normal cycle and early pregnancy. The difficulty of obtaining more precise information on relative potencies in the human has already been stressed.

Mode of action of hormonal contraceptives in women

Most hormonal contraceptives act by suppressing ovulation through the natural feed-back mechanisms which operate between the ovaries, hypothalamus and pituitary during the menstrual cycle. The doses shown in Table VI generally achieve this effect. Although, under certain conditions, oestrogens may stimulate pituitary gonadotrophin production, under other

TABLE VI

EXAMPLES OF DOSES OF SYNTHETIC OESTROGENS AND PROGESTINS USED IN THERAPY

	Dose/day	Use
Diethylstilboestrol	0.1-1 mg	Control of menopausal symptoms
	2-5 mg	Inhibition of ovulation
	10-20 mg	Prostatic & mammary carcinoma therapy
Ethinyloestradiol	0.01-0.05 mg	Control of menopausal symptoms
	0.07 mg	Inhibition of ovulation
Mestranol	0.08 mg	Inhibition of ovulation
Chlormadinone acetate	2 mg with mestranol (0.08 mg) for 5 days after 0.08 mg mestranol for 15 days (Sequens)*	
Medroxyprogesterone acetate	150 mg i.m. every 3 months for contraception	
Dimethisterone	25 mg with ethinyloestradiol (0.1 mg) in Oracon*	
Ethynodiol diacetate	1.0 mg with mestranol (0.1 mg) in Ovulen*	
Norethisterone	1-2 mg with mestranol (0.08-0.1 mg) in ortho-Norvin*	
	10-20 mg daily from 15th to 24th day following oestrogen administration for primary and secondary amenorrhea	
Norethisterone acetate	4 mg with ethinyloestradiol (0.05 mg) in Anovlar 21*	
	3 mg with ethinyloestradiol (0.05 mg) in Gynovlar*	
Norethynodrel	2.5-5 mg with mestranol (0.15-0.075 mg) in Enovid*	
	10 mg with mestranol (0.06 mg) for hypermenorrhoea or endometriosis	
Norgestrel	0.5 mg with ethinyloestradiol (0.05 mg) in Ovral*	

Data mainly from Bingle & Benoit (1973) and from Blacow (1972)

* Oral contraceptive preparation

conditions they are the most powerful inhibitors of pituitary function known. Given alone to suppress ovulation they cause irregular uterine bleeding, and when the medication is stopped ovulation may occur at the time expected for withdrawal bleeding. Progestins alone are weaker and less complete inhibitors of pituitary function, and approximately 50 times the dose is required to obtain equivalent inhibition. Consequently the two hormones are usually given in combination.

Treatment starts on day 5 of the cycle and continues through to day 25; withdrawal bleeding occurs on day 28. Additional contraceptive action is provided by the abnormal responses of the female genital tract to progestin given early in the cycle. For example, progestin inhibits the production of fertile-type cervical mucus and prevents sperm penetration. In the sequential 'pill', first oestrogen alone is given, followed by a combination of oestrogen and progestin; this produces a more normal preparation of the female genital tract, but the effectiveness appears to be lower. In the 'mini-pill', progestin alone is given continuously in small doses which do not usually inhibit ovulation; contraception is achieved by the abnormal effect of continuous progestin action on the genital tract; spotting, or irregular vaginal bleeding, is a common complication.

The combination type of oral contraception abolishes the early rise in FSH and the later peaks of LH and FSH. The sequential 'pill' abolishes both the early and mid-cycle rises in FSH, but aberrant peaks of LH occur during both the administration of oestrogen and of progestin (Swerdloff & Odell, 1969). In the absence of stimulation by FSH, follicles do not develop in the ovaries, and oestrogen and progesterone production remain at uniformly low values.

Metabolism of the sex hormones in the human

The natural steroid hormones are rapidly metabolized and eliminated: oestradiol and progesterone have half-lives of 20 minutes and testosterone one of 11 minutes (Sandberg & Slaunwhite, 1956, 1957, 1958). Some conversions occur peripherally, but the major site of metabolism is the liver. Metabolism occurs by complete reduction of the $\Delta 4-3$ ketone group, common to most of the natural and synthetic hormones except the oestrogens, by oxidation-reduction of hydroxyl and oxo (keto) groups in ring D and by hydroxylation at other sites. Hydroxyl groups are then conjugated with glucuronic acid or sulphuric acid to form water-soluble compounds. Elimination occurs via the kidney, or via the bile and hence into the gut where further modification occurs, and most of the products are reabsorbed into the enterohepatic circulation and ultimately excreted in the urine; small amounts are excreted in the faeces. The main urinary metabolites of oestradiol and oestrone are the conjugates of oestriol, 2-hydroxyoestrone, oestrone, 16-hydroxyoestrone and oestradiol, given in order of decreasing quantitative importance. Approximately 20 other metabolites are eliminated in the urine, which represent stereo-isomers of the main products and of the products of the combinations and permutations of the reactions involved. Oestriol, oestrone and oestradiol (the 'classical' oestrogens) are the metabolites most commonly measured in urine, and these account for approximately 20% of the original oestradiol and oestrone produced. The main urinary metabolite of progesterone is the fully reduced compound, pregnanediol, which accounts for 15% of the progesterone produced (Klopper & Michie, 1956); other products include the partly reduced compound, pregnarolone, and various stereo-isomers of pregnanediol. The main metabolites of testosterone are the two stereo-isomeric oxidation-reduction products, androsterone and aetiocholanolone. The relative proportions of the various metabolites formed from oestradiol and testosterone are influenced by the level of thyroid activity (Gallagher et al., 1960). A minor route for the metabolism of testosterone involves aromatization to oestrogens, and this forms an important source of the oestrogens found in men and in postmenopausal women. This has already been considered (p. 35).

The synthetic steroids are metabolized in the human by the same mechanisms as are the natural compounds. For example, the main metabolites of norethynodrel, ethynodiol diacetate and norgestrel, are the 3α- and 3β-alcohols derived from reduction of the unsaturated structures in ring A, the ethinyl group at position 17 being retained (Cook et al., 1972, 1973; DeJongh et al., 1968). The products are eliminated as the glucuronides and sulphates (Layne et al., 1963). Mestranol is first demethylated to ethinyloestradiol, which circulates in the plasma as the sulphate and is excreted directly in the urine as the glucuronide. The metabolic clearance rates of ethinyloestradiol and of mestranol are similar to that of oestradiol (Bird & Clark, 1973), but the clearance rates of some of the synthetic progestins may be much lower. For example, the metabolic clearance rate of chlormadinone acetate is 127 litres/day, which is less than a tenth that of the natural hormones (Dugwekar et al., 1973).

Diethylstilboestrol is rapidly conjugated in the liver with glucuronic acid; the glucuronide is excreted in the urine or enters the hepatic circulation, and part may be hydrolyzed to the free compound and excreted in the faeces. In the human most of the dose is excreted in the urine, but the faecal route is more important in some animal species (Hanahan et al., 1953).

Just as a small proportion of testosterone is metabolized to oestradiol, so the progestins related to 19-nortestosterone should theoretically be metabolized to ethinyloestradiol or related compounds. Investigation of the urinary metabolites of norethisterone indicated a relatively large (5%) conversion to ethinyloestradiol. This seemed higher than would be expected from the oestrogenic activity of norethisterone, and the possibility was considered that most of the ethinyloestradiol had been produced from a metabolite converted to ethinyloestradiol during the acid hydrolosis which was used in the assay procedure (Brown & Blair, 1960).

Analytical methods

The natural hormones

Bioassay was the original method used for the detection and measurement of the steroid hormones, and it is still used for the evaluation of new or unknown compounds. This was later replaced by chemical analysis of urinary metabolites based on colorimetry. The method of Callow et al. (1938) for the 17-ketosteroid metabolites of the androgens, the method of Brown (1955) for the classical urinary oestrogens and the method of Klopper et al. (1956) for pregnanediol have been widely used. More recently, oestrogen assay by colorimetry has been replaced by fluorimetry based on the Kober-Ittrich procedure (Brown et al., 1968), and better methods for pregnanediol assay have been introduced based on gas-liquid chromatography (GLC) (Cox, 1963). These new urinary methods are in wide-scale, routine, clinical use outside the USA, and fully automated methods have been developed for measuring oestrogens by fluorimetry in the urine of late pregnancy with production rates of 120 analyses per day (Craig et al., 1973). GLC has also been used for measuring oestrogens in urine and plasma (Fischer-Rasmussen, 1972; Morreal et al., 1972).

The most recent advances have involved the use of saturation analysis for the measurement of the very small amounts of hormones in blood. These use either naturally-occurring, specific, binding proteins (competitive protein binding assays), such as uterine cytosol for oestrogens (Korenman et al., 1969) and plasma protein for progesterone and testosterone (Neill et al., 1967; Nugent & Mayes, 1970), or antibodies produced by animals against the steroid conjugated to a protein (radioimmunoassay), such as the method for oestradiol-17β of Abraham (1969). Many such methods have been described during the past 4 years; each has advantages. Uterine cytosol binds oestrogens specifically as a group; this has the advantage of providing a general end-point, and individual oestrogens are separated by various chromatographic procedures. Radioimmunoassay specifically measures substances with closely related structures in unhindered groups and, depending on the specificity of the antiserum, requires less preliminary purification. These new plasma methods have provided the great increase in knowledge on physiological hormone action which has been obtained in the past 6 years.

Rates of hormone production are calculated either by the injection of isotopically-labelled hormone and measurement of the specific activity of a urinary metabolite (Gallagher et al., 1950), or by measurement of the metabolic production rate from a continuous intravenous infusion multiplied by the blood concentration of the hormone. The first method depends on the assumption that a unique metabolite of the hormone can be measured, and in the other the accuracy of the results depends on the constancy of plasma values throughout the day, which cannot be assumed (Tait & Burstein, 1964; Longcope & Tait, 1971).

The synthetic hormones

There are three different circumstances in which measurement of synthetic hormones may be required: the analyst may need to identify or check the amounts of hormones in pharmaceutical preparations or animal feeds, or to measure trace residues in meat or the amounts circulating in plasma or being excreted in the urine.

Diethylstilboestrol

On UV irradiation, diethylstilboestrol (DES) is converted specifically to a yellow product with an absorbance at 418 nm, and this forms the basis of many methods of analysis. Tablets are analyzed after extraction with ethanol-water, and oily solutions after partition between iso-octane and sodium hydroxide (US Pharmacopeia, 1965; Hussey et al., 1973). The reaction was used in the official first-action method of the Association of Official Analytical Chemists for measuring DES in feed pre-mixes and supplements after Soxhlet extraction and solvent partition involving alkali (Horwitz, 1970). A later modification included chromatography on a tripotassium phosphate-celite column and made possible the measurement of 0.55-44 mg DES per kg of feed mix (Jeffus & Kenner, 1972). Schuller (1967) utilized this method for measuring DES in bovine urine. The urine was subjected to hydrolysis and the phenolic fraction was separated by ether extraction and solvent partition with alkali and purified by thin-layer chromatography (TLC) on silica gel. After chromatography the plate was irradiated, and the yellow product was subjected to further chromatography and identified by examination under UV light for absorbance at 254 nm and with fluorescence at 366 nm. The limit of detection was 0.1 µg per sample or 40 µg/l urine.

GLC has also been applied to the measurement of DES in animal foods, using either the free compound or its silyl ethers after simple solvent extraction, with or without further purification (Rutherford, 1970). A method sensitive enough for the measurement of DES residues in various tissues of beef, chicken and lamb was described by Coffin & Pilon (1973). The method involved acetone extraction, acid hydrolysis, solvent partition with alkali, formation of the trifluoro-acetates and gas chromatography using electron capture detection; 2-10 µg/kg could be measured reliably. Two peaks occurred in the chromatograms due to the presence of the cis- and trans- isomers, and this added specificity to the method.

The classical method for detecting DES or other oestrogen additives in food samples specified by the US Code of Federal Regulations (1973) was that of Umberger et al. (1958), based on feeding the samples, mixed with normal feed, to immature female mice and measuring the increase in weight of the uterus; positive reaction indicated that excessive amounts of oestrogens were present in the meat. The method detected 0.8 µg DES/kg. It could also be applied to the detection of oestradiol-17β, with 10 times less sensitivity, and to other oestrogens. Oestrogen feeding could also be detected by examination of prostates of male calves and the genital tracts of heifers receiving the drug (Ruitenberg et al., 1969; Kroes et al., 1970). Radioimmunoassay (RIA) methods for DES have recently been developed, and these are likely to be the preferred methods for detecting specific oestrogens in animal tissues in the future (Abraham et al., 1972). RIA methods are also applicable to oestradiol-17β and its esters occurring in meat (Huis in't Veld et al., 1973).

Ethinyloestradiol, mestranol and progestins

The synthetic steroid hormones can be measured in tablets and in injection fluids by a variety of reactions, including infra-red spectroscopy, UV absorption and various reactions with sulphuric acid or antimony trichloride (US Pharmacopeia, 1965). The British Pharmacopeia (1968) describes a method for the identification and measurement in tablets of 5 synthetic steroid hormones, based on TLC on kieselguhr containing propylene gylcol and visualization of the components by spraying with a sulphuric acid mixture, heating at $110^{\circ}C$ and examination under UV light. Simard & Lodge (1970) describe a similar method, using one-dimensional TLC, for the identification of ethinyloestradiol and mestranol, and using two-dimensional TLC to separate and identify chlormadinone acetate, dimethisterone, ethinyloestradiol, ethynodiol diacetate, mestranol, norethisterone, norethisterone acetate, norethynodrel and norgestrel after extracting the tablets with acetone. Visualization of the separated components by UV light gave a range of detection from 0.1-500 µg, depending on the compound; alternatively, spraying the developed plates with sulphuric acid and heating allowed all the compounds to be detected in amounts of less than 1 µg.

Tissue levels of these synthetic hormones have been assessed in animals and humans by the injection of ^{3}H- or ^{14}C-labelled compounds and the determination of their fate in plasma, tissue and urine (Dugwekar et al., 1973). Radioimmunoassays for these substances are also applicable.

References

Abraham, G.E. (1969) Solid-phase radioimmunoassay of oestradiol-17β. J. clin. Endocr., 29, 866-870

Abraham, G.E., Reifman, E.M., Buster, J.E., Di Stephano, J. & Marshall, J.R. (1972) Production of specific antibodies against diethylstilbestrol. Analyt. Lett., 5, 479-486

Andersen, A.C. (1965) Parameters of mammary gland tumors in aging beagles. J. Amer. vet. med. Ass., 147, 1653-1654

Applezweig, N. (1962) Steroid Drugs, New York, McGraw-Hill

Applezweig, N. (1964) Steroid Drugs, vol. 2, San Francisco, Holden-Day

Baird, D.T., Horton, R., Longcope, C. & Tait, J.F. (1969) Steroid dynamics under steady-state conditions. Recent Progr. Hormone Res., 25, 611-664

Barrett, S.A. & Brown, J.B. (1970) An evaluation of the method of Cox for the rapid analysis of pregnanediol in urine by gas-liquid chromatography. J. Endocr., 47, 471-480

Bingel, A.S. & Benoit, P.S. (1973) Oral contraceptives: Therapeutics versus adverse reactions with an outlook for the future. II. J. pharm. Sci., 62, 349-362

Bird, C.E. & Clark, A.F. (1973) Metabolic clearance rates and metabolism of mestranol and ethynylestradiol in normal young women. J. clin. Endocr., 36, 296-302

Blacow, N.W., ed. (1972) Martindale. The Extra Pharmacopoeia, 26th ed., London, The Pharmaceutical Press

Brazeau, P., Dansereau, M., Gervais, M.H. & Banerjee, R.C. (1973) Hypercoagulabilité sanguine avec administration de norethynodrel: correction par purification de la progestine. Canad. J. Physiol. Pharmacol., 51, 555-558

Breuer, H. (1972) Comparative investigations on the metabolism of steroid hormones in man and animals. In: Plotz, E.J. & Haller, J., eds, Methods in Steroid Toxicology, Los Altos, California, Geron-X

Briggs, M.H. & Brotherton, J. (1970) Steroid Biochemistry and Pharmacology, London, Academic Press

British Pharmacopoeia (1968) London, The Pharmaceutical Press

Brown, J.B. (1955) A chemical method for the determination of oestriol, oestrone and oestradiol in human urine. Biochem. J., 60, 185-193

Brown, J.B. (1957) The relationship between urinary oestrogens and oestrogens produced in the body. J. Endocr., 16, 202-212

Brown, J.B. & Blair, H.A.F. (1960) Urinary oestrogen metabolites of 19-norethisterone and its esters. Proc. roy. Soc. Med., 53, 433

Brown, J.B. & Matthew, G.C. (1962) The application of urinary estrogen measurements to problems in gynecology. Recent Progr. Hormone Res., 18, 337-385

Brown, J.B., MacLeod, S.C., Macnaughtan, C., Smith, M.A. & Smith, B. (1968) A rapid method for estimating oestrogens in urine using a semi-automatic extractor. J. Endocr., 42, 5-15

Callow, N.H., Callow, R.K. & Emmens, C.W. (1938) Colorimetric determination of substances containing the grouping -CH_2CO- in urine extracts as an indication of androgen content. Biochem. J., 32, 1312-1331

Clauberg, C. (1930) Zur Physiologie und Pathologie der sexual Hormone, im besonderen des Hormons des Corpus luteum. I. Der biologische Test für das luteohormon (das spezifische Hormon des Corpus luteum) am infantilen Kaninchen. Zbl. Gynäk., 54, 2757-2770

Coffin, D.E. & Pilon, J.-C. (1973) Gas chromatographic determination of diethylstilbestrol residues in animal tissues. J. Ass. off. analyt. Chem., 56, 352-357

Cook, C.E., Twine, M.E., Tallent, C.R., Wall, M.E. & Bressler, R.C. (1972) Norethynodrel metabolites in human plasma and urine. J. Pharmacol. exp. Ther., 183, 197-205

Cook, C.E., Karim, A., Forth, J., Wall, M.E., Ranney, R.E. & Bressler, R.C. (1973) Ethynodiol diacetate metabolites in human plasma. J. Pharmacol. exp. Ther., 185, 696-702

Cotchin, E. (1962) Problems of comparative oncology with special reference to the veterinary aspects. Bull. Wld Hlth Org., 26, 633-648

Cox, R.I. (1963) Gas chromatography in the analysis of urinary pregnanediol. J. Chromat., 12, 242-245

Craig, A., Leek, J.W. & Palmer, R.F. (1973) An automated method for the determination of estrogens in pregnancy urine. Clin. Biochem., 6, 34-40

DeJongh, D.C., Hribar, J.D., Littleton, P., Fotherby, K., Rees, R.W.A., Shrader, S., Foell, T.J. & Smith, H. (1968) The identification of some human metabolites of norgestrel, a new progestational agent. Steroids, 11, 649-664

Diczfalusy, E. (1969) Steroid metabolism in the human feto-placental unit. Acta Endocr. (Kbh.), 61, 649-664

Dorfman, R.I. (1972) Discussion contribution. In: Plotz, E.J. & Haller, J., eds, *Methods in Steroid Pharmacology*, Los Altos, California, Geron-X

Dugwekar, Y.G., Narula, R.K. & Laumas, K.R. (1973) Disappearance of 1α-^{3}H-chlormadinone acetate from the plasma of women. *Contraception*, 7, 27-45

Elton, R.L. (1959) Metrotropic activity of some 21-haloprogesterone derivatives. *Proc. Soc. exp. Biol.(N.Y.)*, 101, 677-680

Faiman, C. & Ryan, R.J. (1967) Serum follicle-stimulating hormone and luteinizing hormone concentrations during the menstrual cycle as determined by radioimmunoassays. *J. clin. Endocr.*, 27, 1711-1716

Finkel, M.J. & Berliner, V.R. (1973) The extrapolation of experimental findings (animal to man): the dilemma of the systemically administered contraceptives. *Bull. Soc. pharmacol. environm. Path.*, 4, 13-18

Fischer-Rasmussen, W. (1972) Gas-liquid chromatographic measurement of oestriol, oestrone and oestradiol-17β in the plasma of pregnant women. *Dan. med. Bull.*, 19, Suppl. 2, 1-56

Gallagher, T.F., Fukushima, D.K., Barry, M.C. & Dobriner, K. (1950) Studies with isotopic steroid hormones. *Recent Progr. Hormone Res.*, 6, 131-157

Gallagher, T.F., Hellman, L., Bradlow, H.L., Zumoff, B. & Fukushima, D.K. (1960) Effects of thyroid hormones on the metabolism of steroids. *Ann. N.Y. Acad. Sci.*, 86, 605-611

Hanahan, D.J., Daskalakis, E.G., Edwards, T. & Dauben, H.J., Jr (1953) The metabolic pattern of ^{14}C-diethylstilbestrol. *Endocrinology*, 53, 163-170

Horwitz, W., ed. (1970) *Official Methods of Analysis*, 11th ed., Washington DC, Association of Official Analytical Chemists, Secs 38.048-38.051

Huis in't Veld, L.G., Smit, P.J., Kok, G.L., ten Have, T. & Kroonenberg, W.M. (1973) Onderzoek van weefsels van slachtkalveren op residuen van exogene oestrogene stoffen. *Tijdschr. Diergeneesk.*, 98, 749-757

Hussey, R.L., Hale, J.L. & Howard, D.P. (1973) Semiautomated method for determining diethylstilbestrol in low dosage tablet formulations. *J. pharm. Sci.*, 62, 1171-1173

Jeffus, M.T. & Kenner, C.T. (1972) Quantitative determination and confirmation of low levels of diethylstilbestrol in feeds. *J. Ass. off. analyt. Chem.*, 55, 1345-1353

Jenner, M.R., Kelch, R.P., Kaplan, S.L. & Grumbach, M.M. (1972) Hormonal changes in puberty. IV. Plasma estradiol, LH, and FSH in prepubertal children, pubertal females and in precocious puberty, premature thelarche, hypogonadism and in a child with a feminizing ovarian tumor. J. clin. Endocr., 34, 521-530

Jull, J.W. (1973) Ovarian tumorigenesis. In: Busch, H., ed., Methods in Cancer Research, New York, Academic Press, pp. 131-186

Kelch, R.P., Jenner, M.R., Weinstein, R., Kaplan, S.L. & Grumbach, M.M. (1972) Estradiol and testosterone secretion by human, simian and canine testes, in males with hypogonadism and in male pseudohermaphrodites and the feminizing testes syndrome. J. clin. Invest., 51, 824-830

Klopper, A. & Michie, E.A. (1956) The excretion of urinary pregnanediol after the administration of progesterone. J. Endocr., 13, 360-364

Klopper, A., Michie, E.A. & Brown, J.B. (1956) A method for the determination of urinary pregnanediol. J. Endocr., 12, 209-219

Kolb, K.H. (1972) Variations in the pharmacokinetics of sex steroids in laboratory animals. In: Plotz, E.J. & Haller, J., eds, Methods in Steroid Toxicology, Los Altos, California, Geron-X, pp. 92-96

Korenman, S.G. & Sherman, B.M. (1973) Further studies of gonadotrophin and estradiol secretion during the preovulatory phase of the human menstrual cycle. J. clin. Endocr., 36, 1205-1209

Korenman, S.G., Perrin, L.E. & McCallum, T.P. (1969) A radio-ligand binding assay system for estradiol measurement in human plasma. J. clin. Endocr., 29, 879-883

Kroes, R., Ruitenberg, E.J. & Berkvens, J.M. (1970) Histological changes in the genital tract of the female calf after the administration of diethylstilbestrol and hexestrol. Zbl. Vet.-Med., A 17, 440-452

Layne, D.S., Golab, T., Arai, K. & Pincus, G. (1963) The metabolic fate of orally administered ^{3}H-norethynodrel and ^{3}H-norethindrone in humans. Biochem. Pharmacol., 12, 905-911

Lin, T.J., Lin, S.C., Erlenmeyer, F., Kline, I.T., Underwood, R., Billiar, R.B. & Little, B. (1972) Progesterone production rates during the third trimester of pregnancy in normal women, diabetic women and women with abnormal glucose tolerance. J. clin. Endocr., 34, 287-297

Lloyd, C.W., Lobotsky, J., Baird, D.T., McCracken, J.A., Pupkin, M., Zanartu, T. & Puga, J. (1971) Concentrations of unconjugated estrogens, androgens and gestagens in ovarian and peripheral venous plasma of women: the normal menstrual cycle. J. clin. Endocr., 32, 155-166

Longcope, C. (1971) Metabolic clearance and blood production rates of estrogens in postmenopausal women. Amer. J. Obstet. Gynec., 111, 778-781

Longcope, C. & Tait, J.F. (1971) Validity of metabolic clearance and interconversion rates of estrone and 17β-estradiol in normal adults. J. clin. Endocr., 32, 481-490

Longcope, C., Widrich, W. & Sawin, C.T. (1972) The secretion of estrone and estradiol-17β by human testis. Steroids, 20, 439-448

McGinty, D.A., Anderson, L.P. & McCullough, N.B. (1939) Effect of local application of progesterone on the rabbit uterus. Endocrinology, 24, 829-832

McPhail, M.K. (1935) The assay of progestin. J. Physiol. (Lond.), 83, 145-156

Morreal, C.E., Dao, T.L. & Lonergan, P.A. (1972) An improved method for the detection of estrone, estradiol and estriol in low titer urine. Steroids, 20, 383-397

Nandi, S. (1965) Interactions among hormonal, viral and genetic factors in mouse mammary tumorigenesis. Canad. Cancer Conf., 6, 69-81

Neill, J.D., Johansson, E.D.B., Datta, J.K. & Knobil, E. (1967) Relationship between the plasma levels of luteinizing hormone and progesterone during the normal menstrual cycle. J. clin. Endocr., 27, 1167-1173

Nelson, J.H. (1973) Response to Contraception, Philadelphia, Saunders

Nelson, L.W., Weikel, J.H., Jr & Reno, F.E. (1973) Mammary nodules in dogs during four years' treatment with megestrol acetate or chlormadinone acetate. J. nat. Cancer Inst., 512, 1303-1311

Neumann, F. & Elger, W. (1972) Critical considerations of the biological basis of toxicity studies with steroid hormones. In: Plotz, E.J. & Haller, J., eds, Methods in Steroid Toxicology, Los Altos, California, Geron-X, pp. 10-81

Nugent, C.A. & Mayes, D. (1970) Reliability of plasma testosterone assays by competitive protein binding methods. Acta endocr. (Kbh.), 147, Suppl., 257-274

Ross, G.T., Cargille, C.M., Lipsett, M.B., Rayford, P.L., Marshall, J.R., Strott, C.A. & Rodbard, D. (1970) Pituitary and gonadal hormones in women during spontaneous and induced ovulatory cycles. Recent Progr. Hormone Res., 26, 1-62

Ruitenberg, E.J., Kroes, R. & Berkvens, J. (1969) Histological examination of the prostate as a check on oestrogen administration in calves. Zbl. Vet.-Med., B 16, 767-774

Rutherford, B.S. (1970) Gas chromatographic determination of cis- and trans-diethylstilbestrol in feeding pre-mix. J. Ass. off. analyt. Chem., 53, 1242-1243

Sandberg, A.A. & Slaunwhite, W.R., Jr (1956) Metabolism of 4-C^{14}-testosterone in human subjects. I. Distribution in bile, blood, feces and urine. J. clin. Invest., 35, 1331-1339

Sandberg, A.A. & Slaunwhite, W.R., Jr (1957) Studies of phenolic steroids in human subjects. II. The metabolic fate and hepato-biliary-enteric circulation of C^{14}-estrone and C^{14}-estradiol in women. J. clin. Invest., 36, 1266-1278

Sandberg, A.A. & Slaunwhite, W.R., Jr (1958) The metabolic fate of C^{14}-progesterone in human subjects. J. clin. Endocr., 18, 253-265

Schuller, P.L. (1967) Detection of stilboestrol (DES) in urine by thin-layer chromatography. J. Chromat., 31, 237-240

Simard, M.B. & Lodge, B.A. (1970) Thin-layer chromatographic identification of oestrogens and progestins in oral contraceptives. J. Chromat., 51, 517-524

Swerdloff, R.S. & Odell, W.D. (1969) Serum luteinizing and follicle stimulating hormone levels during sequential and non-sequential contraceptive treatment of eugonadal women. J. clin. Endocr., 29, 157-163

Tait, J.F. & Burstein, S. (1964) In vivo studies of steroid dynamics in man. In: Pincus, G., Thimann, K.V. & Astwood, E.B., eds, The Hormones, Vol. 5, New York, London, Academic Press, pp. 441-557

Thomas, K., De Hertogh, R., Pizarro, M., Van Exter, C. & Ferin, J. (1973) Plasma LH-HCG, 17β-estradiol, estrone and progesterone monitoring around ovulation and subsequent nidation. Int. J. Fertil., 18, 65-73

Tulchinsky, D. (1973) Placental secretion of unconjugated estrone, estradiol and estriol into the maternal and the fetal circulation. J. clin. Endocr., 36, 1079-1087

Turner, C.D. & Bagnara, J.T. (1971) General Endocrinology, Philadelphia, Saunders

Umberger, E.J., Gass, G.H. & Curtis, J.M. (1958) Design of a biological assay method for the detection and estimation of estrogenic residues in the edible tissues of domestic animals treated with estrogens. Endocrinology, 63, 806-815

US Code of Federal Regulations (1973) Washington DC, US Government Printing Office, 21 CFR 121.245, 121.257, 135g.30, 135g.38

US Pharmacopeia (1965) 17th Revision, New York, US Pharmacopeial Convention, Inc.

Vallance, D.K. & Capel-Edwards, K. (1971) Chlormadinone and mammary nodules. Brit. med. J., ii, 221-222

Weisburger, J.H. (1968) Hormones, chemicals and liver cancer. N.Z. med. J., 67, 44-58

West, C.D., Mahajan, D.K., Chavré, V.J., Nabors, C.J. & Tyler, F.H. (1973) Simultaneous measurement of multiple plasma steroids by radioimmunoassay demonstrating episodic secretion. J. clin. Endocr., 36, 1230-1236

WHO (1971) Methods of fertility regulation: Advances in research and clinical experience. Wld Hlth Org. techn. Rep. Ser., No. 473

WHO (1973) Advances in methods of fertility regulation. Wld Hlth Org. techn. Rep. Ser., No. 527

OESTROGENS

DIETHYLSTILBOESTROL (STILBOESTROL)

1. Chemical and Physical Data

1.1 Synonyms and trade names*

Chem. Abstr. No.: 56-53-1

DEB; DES; 4,4'-(1,2-diethyl-1,2-ethenediyl)bis-phenol; α,α'-diethylstilbenediol; α,α'-diethyl-4,4'-stilbenediol; trans-α,α'-diethyl-4,4'-stilbenediol; diethylstilbesterol; diethylstilboesterol; trans-diethylstilbesterol; trans-diethylstilboesterol; diethyl-stilbestrol; trans-diethylstilbestrol; trans-diethylstilboestrol; 4,4'-dihydroxy-α,β-diethylstilbene; 3,4-(4,4'-dihydroxyphenyl)hex-3-ene; 3,4-bis(p-hydroxyphenyl)-3-hexene; stilbesterol; stilboesterol; stilbestrol

Bio-des; Climaterine; Comestrol estrobene; Cyren; Cyren A; Cyren B; Di-Estryl; Distilbene; D Oestromon; Domestrol; Estilben; Estilbin MCO; Estril; Estrobene; Estrosyn; Follidiene; Fonatol; Grafestrol; Hi-Bestrol; Idroestril; Microest; Milestrol; Neo-distilbene; Neo-Oestranol; New-Oestranol I; Oestrogenine; Oestromenin; Oestromensil; Oestromensyl; Oestromienin; Oestromon; Palestrol; Percutatrine Oestrogénique Iscovesco; Protectona; Sedestran; Serral; Sexocretin; Sibol; Sintestrol; Stil; Stilbetin; Stilboefral; Stilboestroform; Stilkap; Stil-Rol; Synerstrin; Synestrin; Synthoestrin; Syntofolin

1.2 Chemical formula and molecular weight

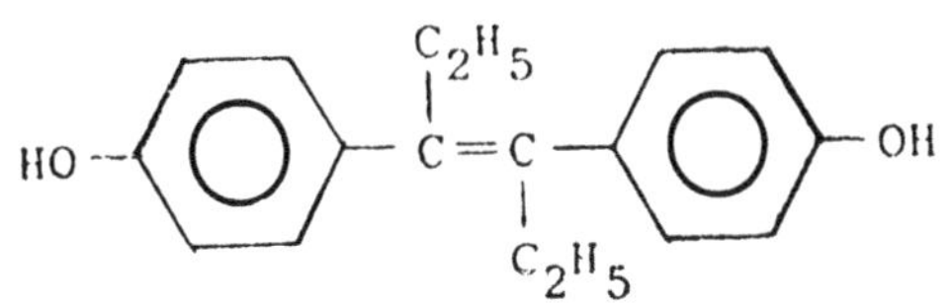

$C_{18}H_{20}O_2$

Mol. wt: 268.3

---

* Trade names include mixtures containing diethylstilboestrol

1.3 Chemical and physical properties of the pure substance

  (a) Description: White platelets (from benzene)
  (b) Melting-point: 169-172°C
  (c) Solubility: Practically insoluble in water; soluble at 25°C in 95% ethanol (1 in 5), chloroform (1 in 200), ether (1 in 3); soluble in acetone, dioxane, ethyl acetate, methyl alcohol, vegetable oils and aqueous solutions of alkali hydroxides.

1.4 Technical products and impurities

The diethylstilboestrol (DES) used commercially is the trans-isomer; the cis-isomer is obtained with difficulty and tends to revert to the trans form (Merck & Co., 1968). DES is available in the United States as a USP grade in tablets, suppositories and in a form suitable for injection. It is also available as the diphosphate ester derivative in the form of tablets and as an aqueous solution of its sodium salt (Kastrup, 1973).

DES was formerly available in the US as implants for use in beef cattle and sheep and as an additive in cattle feeds. Rulings of the US Food and Drug Administration (FDA) have prohibited these uses[1].

2. Production, Use, Occurrence and Analysis

2.1 Production and use[2]

The oestrogenic properties of diethylstilboestrol (DES) were first described by Dodds et al. (1938). A number of synthesis routes have since been developed, all starting with either desoxyanisoin, anisoin, anisole or p-methoxypropiophenone and involving various rearrangements. In a method first reported in 1943, anethole hydrobromide is converted to an intermediate ether using sodamide in liquid ammonia, and this is converted to DES by heating with potassium hydroxide in ethylene gyclol. Commercial

---

[1] A US Court of Appeal, in January 1974, ruled that the FDA had not met all legal requirements in establishing its position. Thus, the legality of the ban has not as yet been resolved.

[2] Data from Chemical Information Services, Stanford Research Institute, USA

production of DES was first reported in the US in 1941, when less than 227 kg were produced (US Tariff Commission, 1945). Although three or more companies have reported production to the US Tariff Commission in several subsequent years, separate data on US production and sales have been published only infrequently. Production data were last reported in 1952, when 1,800 kg were produced (US Tariff Commission, 1953). A total of five US companies are believed to have been producing DES in 1972, but one of these companies has since stopped production. One of the manufacturers also produces the diphosphate ester derivative. Total US sales of DES and its diphosphate ester derivative for use in human medicine are estimated to be less than 500 kg annually.

In 1972, a total of 3,053 kg of DES were reported to have been imported through the principal US customs districts (US Tariff Commission, 1973). This was a sharp reduction from the 5,355 kg reported for 1971 (US Tariff Commission, 1972) and the 5,604 kg reported for 1970 (US Tariff Commission, 1971).

DES is one of the least expensive and most widely used oestrogens. Both DES and its diphosphate ester derivative find use in human medicine for treatment of such conditions as amenorrhea, breast carcinoma, hypogenitalism, menopausal syndrome, postmenopausal oesteoporosis, postpartum breast engorgement, prostatic carcinoma and senile vaginitis. In such applications, DES may be used in combination with androgens and with other medicinals, e.g., vitamins and bactericides (Kastrup, 1972).

In July 1972, as a result of the report of a drug efficacy study group, the FDA concluded that a group of drugs, which included DES vaginal suppositories, were effective in the treatment of post-menopausal and senile vulvovaginitis, atrophic vaginitis, pruritus vulvae caused by atrophic changes in the vulval epithelium, dyspareunia associated with an atrophic vaginal epithelium and for use prior to plastic pelvic surgery in menopausal cases. However, the FDA concluded that there was no substantial evidence of effectiveness if the drug was indicated for mammary hypoplasia. DES has also been used in the past for treatment of threatened abortions, but because of the appearance of genital tract cancers in the female offspring of women who took the drug during their pregnancy (see section 3.3,

"Observations in man", for additional information), new cautions against the use of the drug by pregnant women have been issued (US Environmental Protection Agency, 1972a).

DES has been used in the US in recent years for postcoital contraception, although this application has not been officially approved by the FDA. In September 1973 the FDA, in an effort to restrict the use to emergency treatments only and to discourage its use as a routine method of birth control, announced that new drug applications will be required for this use and that the manufacturers must provide brochures which will explain the risks and benefits of the drug to users (US Environmental Protection Agency, 1973).

Data on production of DES in the countries of Western Europe are not available but production and sales are known to be concentrated in a small number of companies. Total sales of DES in hormone specialties in Western Europe in 1972 are estimated to have been less than 80 kg. Sales in Spain represented approximately 65% of the total, with lesser amounts sold in Belgium, the Federal Republic of Germany, France, Italy, The Netherlands and the United Kingdom.

In the US formerly, DES was implanted (usually in the neck) in male chickens to caponize them chemically and to improve fattening and finishing. The FDA banned such implants in 1959 when residues of DES were found in edible poultry tissue (US Congress, 1973). It was also widely used in the US as a feed additive and as an ear implant to fatten, promote growth and to increase the feed efficiency of beef cattle and sheep. Because of concern about the appearance of residues of DES in food derived from the animals and about the observed carcinogenic properties of DES in test animals, the FDA banned the use of DES in animal feed in August 1972 (US Environmental Protection Agency, 1972b)[1] and banned the use of DES implants on April 27, 1973 (Anon., 1973).

---

[1] A US Court of Appeal, in January 1974, ruled that the FDA had not met all legal requirements in establishing its position. Thus, the legality of the ban has not as yet been resolved.

Veterinary uses of DES include replacement therapy for underdeveloped females, incontinence, vaginitis of spayed bitches, hypertrophy of prostate in dogs and other applications (Merck & Co., 1968). Although no data are available on the quantity of DES consumed in these ways, it is believed that the largest volume used was in feed additives and implants.

In some European countries the use of such oestrogenic hormones as growth promoters in animals is forbidden; in others they are still used.

2.2 Occurrence

Diethylstilboestrol does not occur in nature.

2.3 Analysis

Methods for the analysis of diethylstilboestrol in tablets or feeds are given in the section "General Remarks on the Sex Hormones", p. 42.

3. Biological Data Relevant to the Evaluation of Carcinogenic Risk to Man

3.1 Carcinogenicity and related studies in animals

(a) Oral administration

Mouse: Diethylstilboestrol (DES) when administered in sesame oil by stomach tube produced breast tumours in 18/22 male C3H mice (infected with the mammary tumour virus, MTV) following total doses of 4.25-14.25 mg at the rate of 0.125-0.75 mg twice weekly. The average induction time was 24-28 weeks (Shimkin & Grady, 1941).

Breast tumours were induced in male mice of two hybrid stocks by feeding a semi-synthetic diet containing DES (average intake, 0.5 µg/day/mouse). In intact males the incidences of tumours were lower (11/30 and 12/37) and the average induction times longer (14.6 months and 18.8 months) than in castrates (incidences, 33/34 and 19/20; induction times, 10.7 months and 14.3 months) (Huseby, 1953). Dietary restriction to 1/3 of the caloric intake reduced the breast tumour incidence from 25 to 0% in virgin female A strain mice on a DES-containing diet fed ad libitum. The mammary glands of the restricted mice were considerably less well developed than those of the controls (Ball et al., 1946).

DES was administered in the diet of C3H and A strain mice at levels of 6.25-1000 ppb. At a dose level of 25 ppb the calculated daily intake of DES was 0.06-0.09 µg/mouse, which is comparable to the intake of 0.066 µg found necessary to maintain oestrus. The incidence of breast tumours in virgin female C3H mice maintained on a control diet was 33% (40/121). This incidence was slightly increased with levels of 6.25-25 ppb DES in the diet, and at 50 ppb the incidence was 53% (36/68; P<0.01). With 500 or 1000 ppb, the incidence of breast tumours was more than 84%. The tumour induction times decreased progressively with increased DES concentrations, from 49 weeks on the control diet to 31 weeks at the 1000 ppb dose level. {It is noteworthy that the ovarian weights showed a marked decline with DES concentrations of 25 ppb or more.} Intact male C3H mice only developed a significant incidence of breast tumours (23/60) when 500 ppb DES were given in the diet, although some breast tumours did occur with lower concentrations. Castrated A strain males were less susceptible to all dietary concentrations of DES. No breast tumours occurred in groups of 115 intact male C3H mice or in 136 castrated male A strain controls (Gass et al., 1964).

When DES was given in the diet at levels of 500 and 1000 ppb during 2-, 7-, 14- or 28-day cycles, alternating with similar durations on a control diet, the mammary tumour incidences in groups of castrated male C3H mice were similar in all groups at both dose levels irrespective of the cycle length. However, the incidence of tumours with continuous administration of 250 and 500 ppb DES was significantly higher. Much lower incidences of breast tumours were found in groups of similarly treated intact male mice (Okey & Gass, 1968).

(b) Subcutaneous and/or intramuscular injection

Mouse: Lacassagne (1958) first demonstrated the induction of mammary tumours in 2 male R3 mice following the injection of 25 µg DES twice weekly for 12-16 weeks. Shimkin & Andervont (1942) studied the effects of DES in mice infected with the MTV. Male C3H mice were injected s.c. with DES in sesame oil once a week for 20 weeks (total, 4 mg). In a group suckled by MTV-carrying C3H females, the breast tumour incidence was 9/13 at an average induction time of 9.4 months. C3H males suckled by C57 Black females (without the MTV) had a breast cancer incidence of 2/22, with a latent period of 10.5 months. {Although the MTV was absent in the latter group, the probable presence of the nodule-inducing virus (NIV) must be taken into account in assessing the factors involved in the emergence of mammary tumours (Nandi, 1965).}

Gardner (1959) found neoplastic lesions of the cervix or vagina in 3/14 BC mice injected s.c. weekly with 250 µg DES in sesame oil during 25-41 weeks. {Evaluation of this data is difficult, since the ages of the mice at start of treatment ranged from 26 to 59 weeks.}

Murphy & Sturm (1949) reported a 70% incidence of leukaemia in 40 untreated females of the RIL strain, and untreated males had an incidence of 41% (37/89). In males this was significantly increased to 71% (39/116) by weekly injections of 50 µg DES in oil during 7 months.

Newborn mouse: Dunn & Green (1963) injected newborn male and female mice s.c. with 2 mg DES in saline suspension within the first 24 hours of life. Cancers of the cervix and/or vagina occurred in 6/17 female BALB/c mice aged 13-26 months and in 3/10 C3H females at 20-26 months. Precancerous lesions were found in 3 BALB/c mice at 13-21 months and in 4 female C3H mice at 24-26 months. Granular-cell myoblastomas occurred in 1/6 BALB/c females aged 24-26 months and in 1/9 C3H females at 24-26 months; however, one of these tumours also occurred in 1/2 controls at 26 months. Male mice showed no unusual tumours in any organ.

Hamster: When 0.6 mg DES in 0.2 ml of 0.9% saline was injected s.c. every other day for 36 weeks or longer, 11/16 intact male golden hamsters developed kidney tumours, compared with 0/17 in untreated and 0/5 in saline-treated controls (Kirkman & Bacon, 1952b). {See also under "Subcutaneous implantation".}

Dog: Ovarian lesions were found in all of 8 bitches given s.c. injections of 15-60 mg DES in paraffin oil at 7-8 week intervals during 19 months (total dose, 90-495 mg) (Jabara, 1959). {The identity of these lesions has not been established (O'Shea & Jabara, 1967).}

(c) Subcutaneous implantation (pellets)

Mouse: Pellets (4-6 mg) made from a mixture of cholesterol and amounts of DES ranging from 5 to 50% were implanted into the right axilla in groups of 20-55 male and female strain C mice (Shimkin et al., 1941). Hernias developed in about 10% of males receiving 10-50% DES pellets, and interstitial-cell tumours of the testis were detected between 6 and 11 months in 1/10 mice receiving 5%, in 3/30 receiving 10%, in 4/14 receiving 25% and in 5/8 receiving 50% DES. Three of the tumours metastasized. Mammary tumours occurred in only 1/34 female mice and in 0/20 male mice observed up to 13 months. However, when strain C mice were cross-suckled on C3H mice bearing the MTV, breast tumours occurred between 8 and 11 months in 14/20 females and in 5/13 males implanted with pellets containing 10% DES. Foster nursing did not influence the incidence of testicular tumours, and 2 males had both mammary and testicular tumours. Lymphoid tumours were seen in 4/50 males and in 3/11 females.

In another series of experiments, a high incidence of interstitial-cell tumours of the testis (80%) was found in 76 male mice of the BALB/c strain implanted with 5 mg pellets of 20% DES in cholesterol for "sufficient time for the testes to atrophy" (time not specified). Interstitial-cell tumour induction was found to be dependent on genetic factors, BALB/c being far more susceptible than the RIII, C57BL, C3H, DBA/2, Y and I strains implanted with 10 or 20% DES pellets. Hybridization of males of insusceptible strains with BALB/c females usually, but not invariably, yielded susceptible offspring (0-67% with interstitial-cell tumours) (Andervont et al., 1960).

In experiments to determine whether the susceptibility to interstitial-cell tumours was determined by the genetic constitution of the testis or by some other factor, testes from the susceptible A strain or from the resistant C3H were transplanted to the susceptible F1 hybrid males, which were then implanted with 7 mg pellets containing 25% DES in cholesterol. Tumours arose in a much higher incidence in the transplanted testes from the susceptible A strain, indicating that the site of genetic susceptibility was in the testis itself (Trentin & Gardner, 1958).

In a complex series of experiments Andervont et al. (1957) showed that interruption of exposure to DES for various periods did not affect the induction of testicular tumours. Canter & Shimkin (1968) showed that unilateral orchiectomy significantly reduced the incidences of interstitial-cell tumours, presumably due to reduction of the amount of target tissue. Many DES-induced tumours are dependent on oestrogenic stimulation for continued growth in transplantation (Klein & Hellström, 1962).

When 1.8-2.2 mg pellets of 0.5-30% DES in cholesterol were implanted into male C3H mice which carry the MTV, breast tumours arose in 1/40 (3%) mice bearing pellets containing 0.01 mg DES, and the incidence rose progressively to 87% among 30 mice implanted with pellets containing 0.6 mg DES. The incidence of spontaneous hepatomas was reduced from 26% in untreated males to 9% in males with pellets containing 0.04-0.1 mg DES; there were no hepatomas in mice implanted with 0.2 mg or more DES (Shimkin & Wyman, 1946).

Richardson (1957) reported that the implantation of 7-8 mg pellets of 20% DES in cholesterol increased the incidence and decreased the latent period of breast tumours in virgin hybrid female RIII x C57L mice carrying the MTV. In a group of 48 untreated female mice the incidence was 63% at an average age of 21.3 months; but when the oestrogen pellet was present from 8 weeks of age until death, the incidence of breast tumours in 174 mice rose to 87%, with a mean induction time of 11.1 months. Exposure to DES pellets for periods of 4 or 8 weeks resulted in 75 and 89% incidences and in latent periods of 19.6 and 16.9 months in 40 and 52 mice, respectively.

Experiments intended to determine the carcinogenicity of DES in male mice not carrying the milk-transmitted MTV were carried out using mice which had been freed of the virus by various means. Andervont et al. (1958) reported incidences of mammary cancer varying between 12 and 84% in MTV-free intact or castrated hybrid male or virgin or breeding female mice of the C3H strain and hybrids with BALB/c, RIII and DBA/2 strains. Virgin C3H females and hybrids of C3H with I and C57 mice or crosses between BALB/c, RIII and I and C57 strains treated with DES had less than 10% incidences of breast tumours. The number of mice involved altogether was greater than 2,800. These results are qualified by the fact that although the milk-borne MTV was excluded, the presence of other viruses not transmitted by suckling, such as NIV (Nandi, 1965), cannot be excluded. The differences in tumour incidences in various strains was not, therefore, necessarily due to their differing susceptibilities to DES. The induction of breast tumours in MTV-free male C3H mice was also reported by Heston & Deringer (1953) and by Andervont (1950).

After implantation of cholesterol pellets of approximately 1.6 mg in weight containing 25% DES into virgin female C3H mice (with the MTV), about 0.4 mg of the pellet (equivalent to 0.1 mg DES) was absorbed after one year. On a normal diet, 96% of the mice developed mammary cancer (23/27); however this incidence was reduced to 45% (17/40) when the animals were fed a diet deficient in cystine (White & White, 1944).

In an investigation of the effects of various oestrogens in mice of many strains, Gardner et al. (1944) found that s.c. implants of DES in cholesterol pellets (amounts not clear) increased the incidences of lymphoid tumours in mice of the C3H strain to 26% from 0.3% in untreated controls.

Rat: Initial observations by Geschickter & Byrnes (1942) on the induction of breast tumours by DES in rats were amplified by Dunning et al. (1947). They reported strain differences in susceptibility to breast tumour induction after the s.c. implantation of pellets of DES in cholesterol (1:3) (4-15 mg DES) into 3-4 month-old rats of both sexes. A x C rats had the highest incidence (80% in males, 85% in females); Fischer rats had a lower incidence (22% in males, 17% in females); and the Copenhagen rats developed no breast tumours. Pituitary hypertrophy was least in the Copenhagen strain and greatest in Fischer rats, in which the gland reached weights of 116-155 mg in both females and males. Adrenal cortical tumours occurred in 2 Fischer rats and in 1 A x C rat. Bladder cancers occurred in 22/58 Copenhagen rats and in 3/58 A x C rats, but there were none in Fischer rats. {The occurrence of bladder calculi in all rats with bladder cancer suggests that tumour induction at this site was associated with the formation of bladder stones.}

The incidence of mammary cancer induced by DES treatment was increased by a high-fat diet, but not if the amount of food ingested was restricted isocalorically with controls (Dunning et al., 1949). Changes in the tryptophane content of the diet altered the breast cancer incidence: with 1.4% tryptophane, breast tumours occurred in 100% of rats in a shorter time than they did in rats on control diets (75%) or on diets with 4.3% tryptophane (60%) (Dunning et al., 1950). When the amount of dietary tryptophane was reduced to 0.14%, the incidence of breast tumours was reduced to 56% compared to 85% in controls (Dunning & Curtis, 1954).

Hamster: The induction of malignant adenomatous renal tumours was first described by Kirkman & Bacon (1950) in intact male hamsters implanted with 20 mg pellets of DES for 200 days or longer. In a later study, s.c. implantations of 20 mg pellets of DES (repeated after 200 days) were carcinogenic for the kidney in 52/53 intact male hamsters. Metastases of the kidney tumours were seen in 33/53 animals. Castrated males were equally susceptible as intact males (11/11), and metastases occurred within the abdominal cavity in 3/11 animals. The effective daily dose of DES liberated from pellets was calculated to be 0.09 mg. Intact females were insusceptible to tumour formation (Kirkman & Bacon, 1952a,b). Confirmation and expansion of these results (Horning, 1954, 1956a,b) showed that transplants could be made to hamsters of either sex treated with DES pellets, but that both the primary lesions and the grafts regressed on removal of the oestrogenic stimuli.

Squirrel monkey: Ten adult female squirrel monkeys were implanted s.c. with four 60 mg pellets of DES. In 7/10 animals, malignant uterine mesotheliomas occurred, and in the 3 remaining animals early proliferative lesions of the uterine serosa were observed. Malignant lesions were observed in one animal killed as early as five months after the implantation of DES. Other animals were killed between 11 and 14 months after the initial implantation. No tumours occurred in 4 control animals implanted with cholesterol pellets (McClure & Graham, 1973).

(d) Other experimental systems

Local application: Gardner (1959) found epidermoid carcinomas of the vagina and/or cervix in 3/21 mice of the BC and C57 strains given 1-4 µg DES in oil intravaginally 3 times weekly. Similar lesions occurred in 8/40 BC mice in which pellets of DES in cholesterol (1:3) were fixed in the upper vagina for periods averaging 37 weeks. Vaginal cancers occurred in 1/43 untreated BC mice and in 1/30 BC mice given pellets containing cholesterol only. No vaginal cancers were seen in 11 C57 control mice. {These data are difficult to evaluate because of the advanced age of many of the mice at the start of treatment.}

3.2 Other relevant biological data

See section, "General Remarks on the Sex Hormones", and pp. 38-40.

3.3 Observations in man

Vagina: Adenocarcinoma of the vagina is an extremely rare tumour, especially in young women. In 1971, however, Herbst et al. described 8 patients aged 15-22 years with this condition. An analysis of the previous history of these patients showed that 7 had been born to women who had received DES medication for prior pregnancy loss or for threatened abortion during the relevant pregnancy; none of the mothers of 32 matched control patients had had similar exposure. There were less significant associations with regard to maternal bleeding during the pregnancy and previous foetal loss. These patients were born between 1946 and 1951, which coincides with the time of introduction of DES for the management of high-risk pregnancies (Smith, 1948). Similar data were subsequently reported in smaller numbers of patients by Greenwald et al. (1971, 1973), Henderson et al. (1973), Nissen & Goldstein (1973), Noller et al. (1972), Tsukada et al. (1972) and Williams & Schweitzer (1973).

The vaginal tumours found were mostly clear-cell adenocarcinomas. Accordingly, Herbst and his colleagues established the Registry of Clear-Cell Adenocarcinoma (Mesonephroma) of the Genital Tract in Young Females. Their latest report (Herbst et al., 1972a) includes information concerning 91 patients (53 with vaginal tumours and 38 with cervical tumours). Of the

66 for whom detailed histories were available, 49 had been exposed to synthetic oestrogens in utero; a further 9 had been similarly exposed to unidentified drugs administered because of bleeding or prior pregnancy loss. DES was the drug concerned in 45 cases, dienoestrol in 2, hexoestrol in 1 and DES together with dienoestrol in 1. Details of dosage and duration of DES therapy were available for 46 cases. In all cases the drug was started before the fourth month of pregnancy. The dosage varied widely, the lowest dose being only 1.5 mg per day. Likewise, there was great variation in the duration of therapy: in most cases the drug was given "throughout pregnancy", but in two cases the time of exposure was less than one month. In one, the drug was taken for only 12 days during the first trimester. The patients' ages ranged between 8 and 25 years, and of the 60 whose birthplace had been identified, 57 had been born in various parts of the United States.

The Boston Collaborative Drug Surveillance Program reported by Heinonen (1973) analyzed the data regarding exposure to DES during pregnancy in the period 1959-65 in the 12 centres participating in the United States Collaborative Perinatal Study. A total of 217 DES exposures (almost all of which occurred at two of these centres) was found among the 51,071 pregnancies included in the study. The dose varied widely, from 2.5 to 150 mg/day, with totals of 0.175 to 46.6 g; and the duration of treatment varied from 3 to 212 days. In the same paper, from market research data, it was estimated that the total number of female liveborn offspring exposed to DES in utero during the period 1960-1970 was likely to be between 10,000 and 16,000 per annum in the United States.

Lanier et al. (1973), reviewing case records at the Mayo Clinic, Rochester, identified 818 female infants and 901 male infants born during the interval 1943-59 to mothers who had received some form of oestrogen therapy during pregnancy. In 93% of the pregnancies the oestrogen used was DES. The dosage varied widely, but at that time the recommended dose was usually 5 mg/day, increasing by 5 mg/day every two weeks or every week to 125 mg/day by the 35th week. However, fewer than 4% of the mothers given DES were known to have received a daily dose of 100 mg or more. Follow-up by physical examination or mailed questionnaire was completed to 1970 or later in 99% of cases. No adenocarcinomas of the vagina or cervix were found in any of the young women, and no genito-urinary malignancies were found among the young men.

Carstens & Clemmesen (1972) reported that no cases of adenocarcinoma of the vagina in women under the age of 25 years appeared in the Danish Cancer Registry from 1943 to 1967. Large doses of DES have apparently not been used for the treatment of threatened abortion in that country. According to Ulfelder et al. (1971), no cases of the tumour were found among thousands of patients with gynaecological cancer in the Basel and Frankfurt areas between 1950 and 1970; the use of DES during pregnancy in these areas has also been extremely infrequent. Christine (1971) has reported that no cases of adenocarcinoma of the vagina in women under 25 years of age have appeared in the Connecticut Tumor Registry between 1960 and 1968.

Silverberg & DeGiorgi (1972) have described the structural characteristics of two clear-cell carcinomas of the vagina and discuss the embryological origin of these tumours. They report the observation of 4 cases in all: in 3, the patient's age was between 17 and 22 years and in the fourth, 78. Only one of their patients, aged 17, had a history of in utero exposure to DES.

Herbst et al. (1972b) have detected vaginal adenosis in 13/34 females exposed in utero to DES, and in 7 there were transverse cervical or vaginal ridges. Similar lesions were not present in 275 girls of comparable ages examined consecutively who had no history of DES exposure in utero.

Endometrium: Among 24 female patients with gonadal dysgenesis treated for 5 or more years with DES, endometrial carcinoma developed in 2 and possibly in a third (Cutler et al., 1972). Three such cases had previously been reported by others. Of the total of 5 cases, 3 were of an unusual mixed or adenosquamous type. The average age of the patients was 31 years. It should be noted that the risk of endometrial carcinoma in untreated gonadal dysgenesis is unknown; however, the authors state that the only reported spontaneous endometrial carcinoma occurred in a 79-year old woman.

Breast: There is no evidence that DES is a cause of cancer of the breast in women (see section, "Oestrogens and Progestins in Relation to Human Cancer", p. 227).

According to Campbell & Cummins (1951) and Benson (1957), the great majority of reported cases of breast cancer in men treated with oestrogens for cancer of the prostate are in fact metastases of the prostatic tumour. The report of O'Grady & McDivitt (1969), however, describes a case of primary carcinoma of the breast with Paget's disease of the nipple in a man who had received long-term treatment with DES for carcinoma of the prostate. The most recent paper on this topic (Bülow et al., 1973) reviews 30 cases reported in the world literature between 1946 and 1972. Among the 16 who were treated with DES alone, with total doses varying from 200-44,200 mg, the breast tumour appeared from 1 to 57 months after the start of treatment. On the basis of histological and biochemical investigations, 6 of the tumours were considered to be new primaries and 10 to be metastases.

4. Comments on Data Reported and Evaluation[1]

4.1 Animal data

Diethylstilboestrol (DES) was tested in mice by oral administration, local application and subcutaneous injection, in mice, rats, hamsters and squirrel monkeys by subcutaneous implantation and in hamsters by subcutaneous injection. Its administration to mice resulted in an increased incidence of mammary and lymphoid tumours in both males and females, and of interstitial-cell tumours of the testis in males and cervical and vaginal tumours in females, including those exposed only on the first day of life. In rats, increased incidences of pituitary, mammary and bladder tumours were observed. In hamsters, a high incidence of renal tumours was observed in castrated males and females and in intact males, but not in intact females. In squirrel monkeys, malignant mesotheliomas of the uterine serosa were observed.

DES treatment in most cases increased the incidence of mammary tumours in strains of mice having a spontaneous incidence of these tumours, which may be related to the presence of a virus; testicular tumours occurred in

---

[1] This section should be read in conjunction with the section, "General Conclusions on Hormones", p. 235.

strains having a particular genetic susceptibility to such tumours. No evidence of a possible role of a virus has been shown in rats. Bladder tumours occurred only in rats in which bladder calculi were present.

In most cases, an accurate assessment of the effective carcinogenic dose in implantation studies is not possible. However, in oral administration studies, the lowest statistically significant dose (P<0.01) producing mammary carcinomas in mice was about 0.15 µg/day (6 µg/kg bw/day). This dose is similar to that used in humans in the control of menopausal symptoms by DES (10 µg/kg bw/day) and 30 times less than the dose given for the control of mammary or prostatic cancer (300 µg/kg bw/day).

4.2 Human data

The administration of diethylstilboestrol to women during pregnancy is associated with an increased risk of vaginal or cervical adenocarcinoma in their exposed female offspring. There may also be an increased risk of endometrial carcinoma in women with gonadal dysgenesis treated with this drug. It is possible that the administration of the drug therapeutically to men with carcinoma of the prostate increases the risk of breast cancer.

5. References

Andervont, H.B. (1950) Attempt to detect a mammary tumor agent in strain C mice by estrogenic stimulation. J. nat. Cancer Inst., 11, 73-81

Andervont, H.B., Shimkin, M.B. & Canter, H.Y. (1957) Effect of discontinued estrogenic stimulation upon the development and growth of testicular tumors in mice. J. nat. Cancer Inst., 18, 1-25

Andervont, H.B., Dunn, T.B. & Canter, H.Y. (1958) Susceptibility of agent-free inbred mice and their F1 hybrids to estrogen-induced mammary tumors. J. nat. Cancer Inst., 21, 783-804

Andervont, H.B., Shimkin, M.B. & Canter, H.Y. (1960) Susceptibility of seven inbred strains and the F1 hybrids to estrogen-induced testicular tumors and occurrence of spontaneous testicular tumors in strain BALB/c mice. J. nat. Cancer Inst., 25, 1069-1081

Anon. (1973) DES ban made total by FDA under Delaney Clause rules. Chemical Marketing Reporter, April 30, pp. 4, 25

Ball, Z.B., Huseby, R.A. & Visscher, M.B. (1946) The effect of dietary pseudo-hypophysectomy upon the development of the mammary glands and mammary tumors in mice receiving diethylstilbestrol. Cancer Res., 6, 493

Benson, W.R. (1957) Carcinoma of the prostate with metastases to breasts and testis. Critical review of the literature and report of a case. Cancer, 10, 1235-1245

Bülow, H., Wullstein, H.-K., Böttger, G. & Schröder, F.H. (1973) Mamma-Carcinom bei oestrogenbehandeltem Prostata-Carcinom. Urologe, A 12, 249-253

Campbell, J.H. & Cummins, S.D. (1951) Metastases, simulating mammary cancer, in prostatic carcinoma under estrogenic therapy. Cancer, 4, 303-311

Canter, H.Y. & Shimkin, M.B. (1968) Effect of unilateral orchiectomy on induction of interstitial-cell tumors in BALB/c mice. Cancer Res., 28, 386-387

Carstens, P.H.B. & Clemmesen, J. (1972) Genital-tract cancer in Danish adolescents. New Engl. J. Med., 286, 198

Christine, B. (1971) Adenocarcinoma of vagina: further data. New Engl. J. Med., 285, 524

Cutler, B.S., Forbes, A.P., Ingersoll, F.M. & Scully, R.E. (1972) Endometrial carcinoma after stilbestrol therapy in gonadal dysgenesis. New Engl. J. Med., 287, 628-631

Dodds, E.C., Golberg, L., Lawson, W. & Robinson, R. (1938) Oestrogenic activity of alkylated stilboestrols. Nature (Lond.), 142, 34

Dunn, T.B. & Green, A.W. (1963) Cysts of the epididymis, cancer of the cervix, granular cell myoblastoma and other lesions after estrogen injection in newborn mice. J. nat. Cancer Inst., 31, 425-438

Dunning, W.F. & Curtis, M.R. (1954) Further studies on the relation of dietary tryptophan to the induction of neoplasms in rats. Cancer Res., 14, 299-302

Dunning, W.F., Curtis, M.R. & Segaloff, A. (1947) Strain differences in response to diethylstilbestrol and the induction of mammary gland and bladder cancer in the rat. Cancer Res., 7, 511-521

Dunning, W.F., Curtis, M.R. & Maun, M.E. (1949) The effect of dietary fat and carbohydrate on diethylstilbestrol-induced mammary cancer in rats. Cancer Res., 9, 354-361

Dunning, W.F., Curtis, M.R. & Maun, M.E. (1950) The effect of added dietary tryptophane on the occurrence of diethylstilbestrol-induced mammary cancer in rats. Cancer Res., 10, 319-323

Gardner, W.U. (1959) Carcinoma of the uterine cervix and upper vagina: induction under experimental conditions in mice. Ann. N.Y. Acad. Sci., 75, 543-564

Gardner, W.U., Dougherty, T.F. & Williams, W.L. (1944) Lymphoid tumors in mice receiving steroid hormones. Cancer Res., 4, 73-87

Gass, G.H., Coats, D. & Graham, N. (1964) Carcinogenic dose-response curve to oral diethylstilbestrol. J. nat. Cancer Inst., 33, 971-977

Geschickter, C.F. & Byrnes, E.W. (1942) Factors influencing the development and time of appearance of mammary cancer in the rat in response to estrogen. Arch. Pathol., 33, 334-356

Greenwald, P., Barlow, J.J., Nasca, P.C. & Burnett, W.S. (1971) Vaginal cancer after maternal treatment with synthetic estrogens. New Engl. J. Med., 285, 390-392

Greenwald, P., Nasca, P.C., Burnett, W.S. & Polan, A. (1973) Prenatal stilbestrol experience in mothers of young cancer patients. Cancer, 31, 568-572

Heinonen, O.P. (1973) Diethylstilbestrol in pregnancy. Frequency of exposure and usage patterns. Cancer, 31, 573-577

Henderson, B.E., Benton, B.D.A., Weaver, P.T., Linden, G. & Nolan, J.F. (1973) Stilbestrol and urogenital-tract cancer in adolescents and young adults. New Engl. J. Med., 288, 354

Herbst, A.L., Ulfelder, H. & Poskanzer, D.C. (1971) Adenocarcinoma of the vagina. Association of maternal stilbestrol therapy with tumor appearance in young women. New Engl. J. Med., 284, 878-881

Herbst, A.L., Kurman, R.J., Scully, R.E. & Poskanzer, D.C. (1972a) Clear-cell adenocarcinoma of the genital tract in young females. Registry report. New Engl. J. Med., 287, 1259-1267

Herbst, A.L., Kurman, R.J. & Scully, R.E. (1972b) Vaginal and cervical abnormalities after exposure to stilbestrol in utero. Obstet. Gynec., 40, 287-298

Heston, W.E. & Deringer, M.K. (1953) Occurrence of tumors in agent-free strain $C3H_f$ male mice implanted with estrogen-cholesterol pellets. Proc. Soc. exp. Biol. (N.Y.), 82, 731-734

Horning, E.S. (1954) The influence of unilateral nephrectomy on the development of stilboestrol-induced renal tumours in the male hamster. Brit. J. Cancer, 8, 627-634

Horning, E.S. (1956a) Observations on hormone-dependent renal tumours in the golden hamster. Brit. J. Cancer, 10, 678-687

Horning, E.S. (1956b) Endocrine factors involved in the induction, prevention and transplantation of kidney tumours in the male golden hamster. Z. Krebsforsch., 61, 1-21

Huseby, R.A. (1953) The effect of testicular function upon stilbestrol-induced mammary and pituitary tumors in mice. Proc. Amer. Ass. Cancer Res., 1, 25-26

Jabara, A.G. (1959) Canine ovarian tumours following stilboestrol administration. Austr. J. exp. Biol. med. Sci., 37, 549-566

Kastrup, E.K., ed. (1973) Facts and Comparisons, St. Louis, Missouri, Facts & Comparisons Inc.

Kirkman, H. & Bacon, R.L. (1950) Malignant renal tumours in male hamsters (Cricetus auratus) treated with estrogen. Cancer Res., 10, 122-123

Kirkman, H. & Bacon, R.L. (1952a) Estrogen-induced tumors of the kidney. I. Incidence of renal tumors in intact and gonadectomized male golden hamsters treated with diethylstilbestrol. J. nat. Cancer Inst., 13, 745-752

Kirkman, H. & Bacon, R.L. (1952b) Estrogen-induced tumors of the kidney. II. Effect of dose, administration, type of estrogen and age on the induction of renal tumors in intact male golden hamsters. J. nat. Cancer Inst., 13, 757-765

Klein, G. & Hellström, K.E. (1962) Transplantation studies on estrogen-induced interstitial-cell tumors of testis in mice. J. nat. Cancer Inst., 28, 99-113

Lacassagne, A. (1938) Apparition d'adénocarcinomes mammaires chez des souris males traitées par une substance oestrogène synthétique. C.R. Biol. (Paris), 129, 641-643

Lanier, A.P., Noller, K.L., Decker, D.G., Elveback, L.R. & Kurland, L.T. (1973) Cancer and stilbestrol. A follow-up of 1,719 persons exposed to estrogens in utero and born 1943-1959. Mayo Clinic Proc., 48, 793-799

McClure, H.M. & Graham, C.E. (1973) Malignant uterine mesotheliomas in squirrel monkeys following diethylstilbestrol administration. Lab. Animal Sci., 23, 493-498

Merck & Co. (1968) The Merck Index, Rahway, N.J., pp. 360-361

Murphy, J.B. & Sturm, E. (1949) The effect of diethylstilbestrol on the incidence of leukemia in male mice of the Rockefeller Institute Leukemia strain (R.I.L.). Cancer Res., 9, 88-89

Nandi, S. (1965) Interactions among hormonal, viral and genetic factors in mouse mammary tumorigenesis. Canad. Cancer Conf., 6, 69-81

Nissen, E.D. & Goldstein, A.I. (1973) Stilboestrol therapy in pregnancy. Relationship to vaginal neoplasia in offspring. Nat. Gyn. Obstet., 11, 138

Noller, K.L., Decker, D.G., Lanier, A.P. & Kurland, L.T. (1972) Clear-cell adenocarcinoma of the cervix after maternal treatment with synthetic estrogens. Mayo Clin. Proc., 47, 629-630

O'Grady, W.P. & McDivitt, R.W. (1969) Breast cancer in a man treated with diethylstilbestrol. Arch. Path., 88, 162-165

Okey, A.B. & Gass, G.H. (1968) Continuous versus cyclic estrogen administration: mammary carcinoma in C3H mice. J. nat. Cancer Inst., 40, 225-230

O'Shea, J.D. & Jabara, A.G. (1967) The histogenesis of canine ovarian tumours induced by stilboestrol administration. Path. vet., 4, 137-148

Richardson, F.L. (1957) Incidence of mammary and pituitary tumors in hybrid mice treated with stilbestrol for varying periods. J. nat. Cancer Inst., 18, 813-822

Shimkin, M.B. & Andervont, H.B. (1942) Effect of foster nursing on the induction of mammary and testicular tumors in mice injected with stilbestrol. J. nat. Cancer Inst., 2, 611-622

Shimkin, M.B. & Grady, H.G. (1941) Toxic and carcinogenic effects of stilbestrol in strain C3H male mice. J. nat. Cancer Inst., 2, 55-60

Shimkin, M.B. & Wyman, R.S. (1946) Mammary tumors in male mice implanted with estrogen-cholesterol pellets. J. nat. Cancer Inst., 7, 71-75

Shimkin, M.B., Grady, H.G. & Andervont, H.B. (1941) Induction of testicular tumors and other effects of stilbestrol-cholesterol pellets in strain C mice. J. nat. Cancer Inst., 2, 65-80

Silverberg, S.G. & DeGiorgi, L.S. (1972) Clear-cell carcinoma of the vagina. A clinical, pathologic and electron microscopic study. Cancer, 29, 1680-1690

Smith, O.W. (1948) Diethylstilbestrol in the prevention and treatment of complications of pregnancy. Amer. J. Obstet. Gynec., 56, 821-834

Trentin, J.J. & Gardner, W.U. (1958) Site of gene action in susceptibility to estrogen-induced testicular interstitial-cell tumors of mice. Cancer Res., 18, 110-112

Tsukada, Y., Hewett, W.J., Barlow, J.J. & Pickren, J.W. (1972) Clear-cell adenocarcinoma ("mesonephroma") of the vagina. Three cases associated with maternal synthetic nonsteroid estrogen therapy. Cancer, 29, 1208-1214

Ulfelder, H., Poskanzer, D. & Herbst, A.L. (1971) Stilbestrol-adenosis-carcinoma syndrome: geographic distribution. New Engl. J. Med., 285, 691

US Congress (1973) Regulation of diethylstilbesterol (DES) and other drugs used in food producing animals. Union Calendar No. 315, House Report No. 93-708, Washington DC, US Government Printing Office, pp. 6, 7, 18, 44, 45, 46

US Environmental Protection Agency (1972a) Drugs for human use; drug efficacy study implementation. US Federal Register, 37, Washington DC, US Government Printing Office, pp. 15028-15029

US Environmental Protection Agency (1972b) Diethylstilbestrol. Order denying hearing and withdrawing approval of new animal drug applications for liquid and dry premixes, and deferring ruling on implants. US Federal Register, 37, Washington DC, US Government Printing Office, p. 15747

US Environmental Protection Agency (1973) Diethylstilbestrol. Use as a postcoital contraceptive; patients labeling. US Federal Register, 38, No. 186, Washington DC, US Government Printing Office, pp. 26809-26811

US Tariff Commission (1945) Synthetic Organic Chemicals, US Production and Sales 1941-43, Second Series, Report No. 153, Washington DC, US Government Printing Office, p. 41

US Tariff Commission (1953) Synthetic Organic Chemicals, US Production and Sales 1952, Second Series, Report No. 190, Washington DC, US Government Printing Office, p. 33

US Tariff Commission (1971) Imports of Benzenoid Chemicals and Products 1970, TC Publication 413, Washington DC, US Government Printing Office, p. 82

US Tariff Commission (1972) Imports of Benzenoid Chemicals and Products 1971, TC Publication 496, Washington DC, US Government Printing Office, p. 86

US Tariff Commission (1973) Import of Benzenoid Chemicals and Products 1972, TC Publication 601, Washington DC, US Government Printing Office, p. 85

White, F.R. & White, J. (1944) Effect of diethylstilbestrol on mammary tumor formation in strain C3H mice fed a low cystine diet. J. nat. Cancer Inst., 4, 413-415

Williams, R.R. & Schweitzer, R.J. (1973) Clear-cell adenocarcinoma of the vagina in a girl whose mother had taken diethylstilbestrol. Calif. Med., 118, 53-55

ETHINYLOESTRADIOL

1. Chemical and Physical Data

1.1 Synonyms and trade names*

Chem. Abstr. No.: 57-63-6

3,17β-Dihydroxy-17α-ethynyl-1,3,5(10)-estratriene; 3,17β-dihydroxy-17α-ethynyl-1,3,5(10)-oestratriene; 17α-ethinyl-3,17-dihydroxy-$\Delta^{1,3,5}$-estratriene; 17α-ethinyl-3,17-dihydroxy-$\Delta^{1,3,5}$-oestratriene; ethinyl estradiol; ethinyl oestradiol; 17-ethinyl estradiol; 17-ethinyl oestradiol; 17-ethinyl-3,17-estradiol; 17-ethinyl-3,17-oestradiol; 17α-ethinylestradiol; 17α-ethinyloestradiol; 17α-ethinyl-$\Delta^{1,3,5(10)}$-estratriene-3,17β-diol; 17α-ethinyl-$\Delta^{1,3,5(10)}$-oestratriene-3,17β-diol; 17α-ethinylestra-1,3,5(10)-triene-3,17β-diol; 17α-ethinyloestra-1,3,5(10)-triene-3,17β-diol; 17-ethynyl-estradiol; 17-ethynyloestradiol; 17α-ethynylestradiol; 17α-ethynyl-oestradiol; 17α-ethynylestradiol-17β; 17α-ethynyloestradiol-17β; 17α-ethynyl-17β-estradiol; 17α-ethynyl-17β-oestradiol; 17-ethynyl-estra-1,3,5(10)-triene-3,17β-diol; 17-ethynyloestra-1,3,5(10)-triene-3,17β-diol; 17α-ethynyl-1,3,5-estratriene-3,17β-diol; 17α-ethynyl-1,3,5-oestratriene-3,17β-diol; 17α-ethynylestra-1,3,5(10)-triene-3,17β-diol; 17α-ethynyloestra-1,3,5(10)-triene-3,17β-diol; 19-nor-17α-pregna-1,3,5(10)-trien-20-yne-3,17-diol; (17α)-19-norpregna-1,3,5(10)-trien-20-yne-3,17-diol

Amenoron; Amenorone; Anovlar; Anovlar 21; Anovlar Mite; Ciclo Complex; Controvlar; Delpregnin; Demulen 50; Dimenoral; Diognat-E; Diogyn-E; Dipro; Distilbene; Duogynon; Duogynon Oral; Duoluton; Dyloform; EE; Estandron; Esteed; Estigyn; Estinyl; Eston-E; Estoral (Orion); Estrovister; Etalontin; Etalontin 28; Ethidol; Ethinoral; Ethinyl-oestranol; Ethy 11; Eticyclin; Eticyclol; Etinestrol; Etinestryl; Etinilestrad; Etinoestryl; Etivex;

---

* Trade names include mixtures containing ethinyloestradiol

Eugynon; Eugynon 21; Eugynon 28; Eugynon ED; Evanor; Folinett; Follinyl; Gestovex; Gineserpina; Ginestrene; Gynostat; Gynovlane; Gynovlar; Gynovlar 21; Hormoduvadilan; Inestra; Kombikwens; Kombiquens; Kolpolyn; Linoral; Lutestral; Lutogynoestryl; Lutogynoestryl Fort; Lynoral; Menokwens; Menolyn; Menopax; Menoquens; Menstrogen; Menstrogon; Metrulen; Milli-Anovlar; Minilyn; Minovlar; Minovlar ED; Neo-Delpregnin; Neo-Estrone; Neogentrol; Neogynon; Neogynon ED; Neogynon 21; Neogynon 28; Neovlar 21; Neovulen; N Gestakliman; Nordiol 21; Nordiol 28; Norlestrin; Norlestrin 21; Norquentiel; Novestrol; Novokwens; Nuvacon; Oestradin; Oracon; Oraconal; Oradiol; Orestralyn; Orlest; Orlest 28; Ovin; Ovisec; Ovral; Ovran; Ovulen; Ovulen 1/50; Ovulen 50; Ovulene 50; Palonyl; Perovex; Piloval; Planor; Planovin; Primodian; Primodos; Primogyn; Primogyn C; Primogyn M; Primosiston; Primovlar 21; Primovlar 28; Prociclo; Profinix; Progylut; Progynon C; Progynon M; Protex; Pseudosolasodine B; Reglovis; Salvacal; Secrodyl; Secrovin; Serial; Serial 4x7; Serial 28; Serial C; Stediril; Stediril D; Synchron; Tova; Verafem; Volidan; Volidan 21; Volidan V; Volplan; Voplan

1.2 <u>Chemical formula and molecular weight</u>

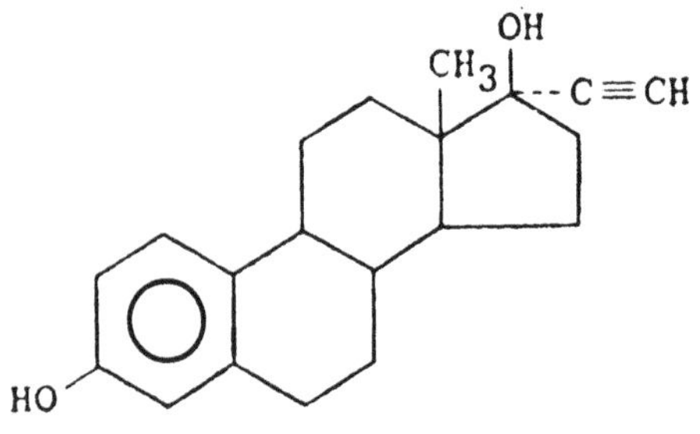

$C_{20}H_{24}O_2$

Mol. wt: 296.4

1.3 Chemical and physical properties of the pure substance

(a) Description: Fine white needles (from methanol and water)

(b) Melting-point: 182-184°C (when freshly crystallized it also occurs in a less stable form with a melting-point of 141-146°C)

(c) Absorption spectrometry: λ_{max} 248 nm

(d) Optical rotation: $\{\alpha\}_D^{25}$ +1° to +10° (10% w/v in dioxane)

(e) Solubility: Practically insoluble in water; soluble at 25°C in 95% ethanol (1 in 6), acetone (1 in 5), chloroform (1 in 20), dioxane (1 in 4), ether (1 in 4), vegetable oils and aqueous solutions of alkali hydroxides

1.4 Technical products and impurities

In the United States ethinyloestradiol is available as a USP grade in the form of tablets. It is also available in several combinations with progestins for uses such as oral contraception and pregnancy testing (Kastrup, 1973).

2. Production, Use, Occurrence and Analysis

2.1 Production and use[1]

The synthesis of ethinyloestradiol was first reported by Inhoffen et al. (1938). It is not produced commercially in the US, but it is believed to be made commercially in other countries by the treatment of oestrone with potassium acetylide in liquid ammonia.

Ethinyloestradiol is one of the most active steroid oestrogens known. It is used in human medicine for the treatment of such conditions as amenorrhea, breast carcinoma, hypogonadism, menopausal disorders, post-partum breast engorgement and prostatic carcinoma. In such applications it is sometimes used in combination with androgens or with progestins

---

[1] Data from Chemical Information Services, Stanford Research Institute, USA

(e.g., for pregnancy testing). However, by far the most widespread use of ethinyloestradiol is in oral contraceptives. It is used as the oestrogen in progestin-oestrogen combination therapy and as both the active ingredient in the oestrogen tablet and the oestrogen component of progestin-oestrogen tablets used in sequential therapy (Kastrup, 1973). Total US sales of ethinyloestradiol for use in human medicine are estimated to be less than 50 kg annually.

Data on production of ethinyloestradiol in the countries of Western Europe are not available, but it is believed to be produced by at least one producer in each of the following countries: the Federal Republic of Germany, France, Italy, The Netherlands and the United Kingdom. Total sales of ethinyloestradiol in hormone and contraceptive specialties in Western Europe in 1972 are estimated to have been less than 100 kg. Sales in Belgium represented approximately 35% of the total, with lesser amounts sold in the Federal Republic of Germany, France, Italy, The Netherlands, Spain and the United Kingdom.

Ethinyloestradiol is not used as a growth promoter in animals. Its veterinary applications are similar to those of oestradiol, e.g., in replacement therapy in underdeveloped females, in the treatment of incontinence and vaginitis in spayed bitches and in the treatment of various reproductive disorders (Merck & Co., 1968).

2.2 Occurrence

Ethinyloestradiol does not occur in nature.

2.3 Analysis

General methods of analysis are summarized in the section, "General Remarks on the Sex Hormones", p. 43.

3. Biological Data Relevant to the Evaluation of Carcinogenic Risk to Man

3.1 Carcinogenicity and related studies in animals

Since only a few studies have been made on ethinyloestradiol alone, most information has been derived from studies made with combinations with progestins. The experimental data have therefore been summarized both under "ethinyloestradiol" and under the other compounds used in these combinations. It is important to note that the effects reported may therefore reflect the action of an individual constituent or of the combination.

(a) Oral administration

Mouse: Poel (1966) administered 7 or 70 µg of a mixture of norethisterone plus ethinyloestradiol (50:1) in oil by gavage, 5 times per week, to groups of 24 virgin female C57L mice, commencing when the animals were 13 weeks of age. Pituitary tumours were present at autopsy after 84 weeks of treatment in 7/15 surviving mice given the lower dose and in 5/8 mice given the higher dose. Pituitary tumours were observed in 2/15 controls. Hepatomas were found in 10/96 mice initially treated with norethisterone plus ethinyloestradiol or with norethynodrel plus mestranol, but the report does not specify in which group or groups they arose. No hepatomas occurred in 48 controls.

The Committee on Safety of Medicines (1972) coordinated a trial of ethinyloestradiol alone or in combination with ethynodiol diacetate, norethisterone acetate, norgestrel or megestrol acetate. The drugs were evaluated for carcinogenicity by incorporation in the diet of 2 strains of mice (CF-LP and BDH) for 80 weeks. The doses were identified only as low (2-5 times the human dose), medium (50-150 times) or high (200-400 times). The amounts administered were not specified.

Ethinyloestradiol administered alone increased the incidence of pituitary tumours in both male and female CF-LP mice in one of two experiments in 2-8/120 to 26-38/120 mice. Similar increases were found with ethinyloestradiol in combination with ethynodiol diacetate or norethisterone acetate but not with norgestrel. {The negative findings in one group on ethinyloestradiol alone and in one group administered ethinyloestradiol plus norgestrel may have been due to undetected differences in the conduct of the trial.} Malignant tumours of the connective tissue of the uterus (unspecified) were found in 6/120 female mice fed ethinyloestradiol plus ethynodiol diacetate compared with 0-1/120 controls.

In groups of 71-87 mice of the BDH-SPF Carshalton stock, administration of ethinyloestradiol alone or in combination with megestrol acetate was associated with a small increase in the incidence of pituitary tumours in treated males and females (4-10% in treated groups compared with 2 and 0% in 57 male and 65 female controls); benign gonadal tumours (unspecified) were found in males (8-10% compared with 0% in controls); incidences of malignant mammary tumours were increased in both males and females (9-32% compared with 0% and 3% in controls); malignant tumours of the uterine fundus and of the cervix were found in 4-11% and in 4%, respectively, of the female treatment groups compared with 0% in female controls.

Lutestral (97.5% chlormadinone acetate and 2.5% ethinyloestradiol), when fed in the diet at 8 ppm (daily intake, 20-30 μg/mouse) altered neither the breast tumour incidence nor the latent period in intact female RIII, C3H or (C3H x RIII)F_1 mice. In intact male (C3H x RIII)F_1 mice the tumour incidence was increased from 0% to 31% (0/76 and 10/32) and in castrated male (C3H x RIII)F_1 mice from 33% to 78% (20/61 and 23/28) with a decrease in the latent period (Rudali, 1974).

Rat: McKinney et al. (1968) reported that in groups of 30 female Mead-Johnson rats, administration of ethinyloestradiol in the diet, either alone at an average dose of 53 μg/kg bw/day or at the same dose level with megestrol acetate (average, 2.63 mg/kg bw/day), for 104 weeks did not increase the incidence of tumours in any tissue. When ethinyloestradiol (30 μg/kg bw/day) was given for 16 days followed by a mixture of ethinyloestradiol (30 μg/kg bw/day) plus megestrol acetate (1.5 mg/kg bw/day) for 5 days and then a period of no steroid treatment for 7 days, for a total of 26 cycles (104 weeks), there was a significant reduction in the incidence of mammary tumours compared with that in controls.

The Committee on Safety of Medicines (1972) (see under "mouse" for details) reported differences between control (24-100 rats/group) and test groups (72-120 rats/group) given ethinyloestradiol alone or in combination with ethynodiol diacetate, norethisterone acetate, norgestrel or megestrol acetate for 104 weeks. Benign mammary tumours were found more frequently in males given the combination with norethisterone acetate (28% compared with 2% in controls), and malignant mammary tumours were found more frequently in males given the combination with ethynodiol diacetate (10% compared with 0% in controls). The incidence of benign liver-cell tumours was increased in males and females given ethinyloestradiol alone (15 and 23%) or in combination with megestrol acetate (11 and 14%) compared with 0 and 8% in male and female controls. In females, the incidence of malignant liver-cell tumours in groups treated with ethinyloestradiol alone or in combinations ranged from 3% for ethinyloestradiol plus megestrol acetate (1:5) to 8% for ethinyloestradiol alone, a very significant finding compared with the virtual absence of such lesions in 12 separate control groups of female rats.

(b) Subcutaneous and/or intramuscular injection

Rat: Hisamatsu (1972) injected small groups of 10 female Wistar rats s.c. with 5, 10 or 15 mg/kg bw of a mixture of ethinyloestradiol with megestrol acetate (1:8) in olive oil once every other day for 1 month. Mammary fibroadenomas occurred in 8/27 survivors between 29 and 59 weeks compared with 0/10 surviving controls.

3.2 Other relevant biological data

See section, "General Remarks on the Sex Hormones", and pp. 38-40.

3.3 Observations in man

See section, "Oestrogens and Progestins in Relation to Human Cancer", p. 219.

4. Comments on Data Reported and Evaluation[1]

4.1 Animal data

Ethinyloestradiol was tested in mice and rats by the oral route; in most cases it was administered in combination with progestins. Administered alone to mice, it increased the incidence of pituitary tumours and malignant mammary tumours in both males and females and produced malignant

---

[1] This section should be read in conjunction with the section, "General Conclusions on Hormones", p. 235.

tumours of the uterine fundus and the cervix in females. In rats, it increased the incidence of benign liver-cell tumours in both males and females and produced malignant liver-cell tumours in females.

When ethinyloestradiol was given in combination with some progestins, excess incidences of malignant tumours of the uterine fundus in female mice and of benign and/or malignant mammary tumours in male rats were observed; in female rats the combinations reduced but did not prevent the incidence of malignant liver-cell tumours when compared with that produced by ethinyloestradiol alone.

Mammary fibroadenomas were produced in female rats following subcutaneous injection of a combination of ethinyloestradiol with a progestin.

4.2 Human data

No case reports or epidemiological studies on ethinyloestradiol alone were available to the Working Group. Epidemiological studies on steroid hormones used in oestrogen-progestin contraceptive preparations have been summarized in the section, "Oestrogens and Progestins in Relation to Human Cancer", p. 223.

5. References

Committee on Safety of Medicines (1972) *Carcinogenicity tests of oral contraceptives*, London, HMSO

Hisamatsu, T. (1972) Mammary tumorigenesis by subcutaneous administration of a mixture of megestrol acetate and ethynylestradiol in Wistar rats. *Gann*, 63, 483-485

Inhoffen, H.H., Logemann, W., Hohlweg, W. & Serini, A. (1938) Untersuchungen in der sexual Hormon-Reihe. *Ber. dtsch. chem. Ges.*, 71, 1024-1033

Kastrup, E.K., ed. (1973) *Facts and Comparisons*, St. Louis, Missouri, Facts & Comparisons Inc.

McKinney, G.R., Weikel, J.H., Jr, Webb, W.K. & Dick, R.G. (1968) Use of the life-table technique to estimate effects of certain steroids on probability of tumor formation in a long-term study in rats. *Toxicol. appl. Pharmacol.*, 12, 68-79

Merck & Co. (1968) *The Merck Index*, 8th ed., Rahway, N.J., p. 423

Poel, W.E. (1966) Pituitary tumors in mice after prolonged feeding of synthetic progestins. *Science*, 154, 402-403

Rudali, G. (1974) Induction of tumors in mice with synthetic sex hormones. *Gann Monograph* (in press)

MESTRANOL

1. Chemical and Physical Data

1.1 Synonyms and trade names*

Chem. Abstr. No.: 72-33-3

Compound 33355; EE3ME; 17α-ethinyl estradiol 3-methyl ether; 17α-ethinyl oestradiol 3-methyl ether; ethinylestradiol 3-methyl ether; ethinyloestratiol 3-methyl ether; ethinylestradiol methyl ether; ethinyloestradiol methyl ether; ethynylestradiol 3-methyl ether; ethynyloestradiol 3-methyl ether; 17α-ethynylestradiol 3-methyl ether; 17α-ethynyloestradiol 3-methyl ether; 17α-ethynylestradiol methyl ether; 17α- ethynyloestradiol methyl ether; (+)-17α-ethynyl-17β-hydroxy-3-methoxy-1,3,5(10)-estratriene; (+)-17α-ethynyl-17β-hydroxy-3-methoxy-1,3,5(10)-oestratriene; 17-ethynyl-3-methoxy-1,3,5(10)-estratrien-17β-ol; 17-ethynyl-3-methoxy-1,3,5(10)-oestratrien-17β-ol; 17α-ethynyl-3-methoxy-17β-hydroxy-$\Delta^{1,3,5(10)}$-estratriene; 17α-ethynyl-3-methoxy-17β-hydroxy-$\Delta^{1,3,5(10)}$-oestratriene; 3-methoxy-17α-ethinyl-estradiol; 3-methoxy-17α-ethinyloestradiol; 3-methoxyethynylestradiol; 3-methoxyethynyloestradiol; 3-methoxy-17α-ethynylestradiol; 3-methoxy-17α-ethynyloestradiol; 3-methoxy-17α-ethynyl-1,3,5(10)-estratrien-17β-ol; 3-methoxy-17α-ethynyl-1,3,5(10)-oestratrien-17β-ol; 3-methoxy-19-nor-17α-pregna-1,3,5(10)-trien-20-yn-17-ol; 19-nor-17α-pregna-1,3,5(10)-trien-20-yn-17-ol, 3-methoxy-; 3-methoxy-(17α)-19-norpregna-1,3,5(10)-trien-20-yn-17-ol; 3-methoxy-19-nor-17α-pregna-1,3,5(10)-trien-20-yn-17β-ol; delta-MVE; SC 4725

Aconcen; Anacyclin; Anconcene; Conlunett; Conlunett 21; Conluten; Conovid; Conovid E; Consan; C-Quens; C-Quens-21; Cyclovul; Delpregnin; Demulen; Enavid; Enavid E; Enovid; Enovid E; Estirona; Estirona 21; Eunomin; Feminor 21; Feminor Seq.; Gestakliman;

---

* Trade names include mixtures containing mestranol

Gynovin; Hestranol; Inostral; Luteolas; Lynacyclan; Lyndiol; Lyndiol Mite; Lyndiol 2.5; Lyndiol-22; Mestrenol; Metrulen; Metrulen M; Metrulene; Neonovum; Nocon; Nonovul; Nor 50; Noracyclin; Noracyclin 22; Noracycline 22; Norinyl; Norinyl 1; Norinyl 1/28; Norinyl 2; Norolen; Nuriphasic; Orgaluton; Ortho-Novin; Ortho-Novin Sq.; Ortho-Novin 2; Ortho-Novin 1/50; Ortho-Novin 1/80; Ortho-Novin Mite; Orthonovum; Orthonovum N; Ortho-Novum; Ortho-Novum Sq.; Ortho-Novum 1/50; Ortho-Novum 1/80; Ortho-Novum 2; OV 28; Ovanon; Ovariostat; Ovostat; Ovulen; Ovulen 0.5; Ovulen 1; Ovulen Mite; Plan; Previsan; Previsana; Sequens; Singestol; Singestrol; Sistometril; Volenyl

1.2 Chemical formula and molecular weight

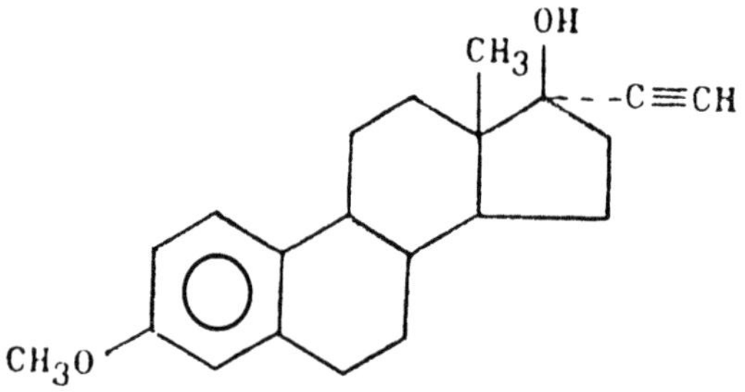

$C_{21}H_{26}O_2$

Mol. wt: 310.4

1.3 Chemical and physical properties of the pure substance

(a) *Description*: White crystals (from methanol or acetone)
(b) *Melting-point*: 150-151°C
(c) *Solubility*: Slightly soluble in water; soluble at 25°C in 95% ethanol (1 in 44), acetone and ether (1 in 23), chloroform (1 in 4.5), dioxane (1 in 12) and methanol

1.4 Technical products and impurities

Mestranol is available in the United States only in combinations with other oestrogens and progestins for use in, for example, oral contraception and treatment of menstrual disorders (Kastrup, 1973). Mestranol is present at levels up to 1% in norethynodrel as normally manufactured (Blacow, 1972).

2. Production, Use, Occurrence and Analysis

2.1 Production and use[1]

Although the US patent 2,666,769 was granted to F.B. Colton in 1954, this chemical is not produced commercially in the US at present. It is believed to be made commercially in other countries by treatment of oestrone 3-methyl ether with potassium acetylide in liquid ammonia.

Mestranol is used in human medicine in combination with a progestin for the treatment of such conditions as endometriosis and hypermenorrhea. However, by far the most widespread use for mestranol is in oral contraceptives where it is used as the oestrogen in progestin-oestrogen combination therapy and as both the active ingredient in the oestrogen tablet and the oestrogen component of progestin-oestrogen tablets used in sequential therapy (Kastrup, 1973). Total US sales of mestranol for use in human medicine are estimated to be less than 100 kg annually. As far as is known, mestranol is not used in veterinary medicine.

Data concerning production of mestranol in the countries of Western Europe are not available, but production and sales are known to be concentrated in a small number of companies. Total sales of mestranol in hormone and contraceptive specialties in Western Europe in 1972 are estimated to have been less than 70 kg. Sales in the United Kingdom represented approximately 65% of the total, with lesser amounts sold in the Federal Republic of Germany, France, Italy and The Netherlands.

2.2 Occurrence

Mestranol does not occur in nature.

2.3 Analysis

General methods of analysis are summarized in the section, "General Remarks on Sex Hormones", p. 43.

---

[1] Data from Chemical Information Services, Stanford Research Institute, USA

3. Biological Data Relevant to the Evaluation of Carcinogenic Risk to Man

3.1 Carcinogenicity and related studies in animals

In several of the following investigations, mestranol was administered as the commercial product "Enovid" (1.5% mestranol and 98.5% norethynodrel), or in combination with other progestins. The experimental data has therefore been summarized under both "mestranol" and "norethynodrel", and it should be noted that the results reported may reflect the action either of the constituent drug alone or of the combination.

(a) Oral administration

Mouse: Poel (1966) administered 7 or 70 µg of a mixture of mestranol: norethynodrel (1:50) in oil by gavage 5 times per week to groups of 24 virgin female C57L mice. Pituitary tumours were present at autopsy in 7/7 mice surviving 84-89 weeks at the higher dose level and in 6/11 mice at the lower dose level, compared with 2/15 controls surviving 90 weeks. In this, and in a concurrent experiment with norethisterone and ethinyloestradiol, hepatomas were found in 10/96 of the C57L mice initially used, but the distribution within the different treatment groups was not reported. No hepatomas occurred among 48 control mice.

Dunn (1969) fed a liquid diet (Metrecal) containing Enovid to female BALB/c mice and estimated that each mouse consumed 10-12.5 µg of the drug per day. All of the 8 mice surviving more than 74 weeks of treatment had early or infiltrating carcinoma of the cervix. No carcinomas of the uterus, cervix or vagina were found in 42 untreated females surviving 103-130 weeks nor in 8 females on Metrecal for 79-102 weeks.

Enovid added to the diet at 15 ppm (average intake, 30-40 µg/mouse/day) increased the mammary tumour incidence in castrated male (C3H x RIII)F_1 mice from 16 to 87% (10/61 and 20/23). The latent period for tumour development was decreased in both castrated males and ovariectomized females, but the incidence in ovariectomized females was not significantly increased. In intact female RIII mice Enovid had no effect on incidence or on latent period (Rudali, 1974).

Ovulen (90% ethynodiol diacetate and 10% mestranol) mixed in the diet at 3 ppm (intake, 7.5-10.0 µg/mouse/day) increased the incidence of breast tumours in intact male (C3H x RIII)F_1 mice from 0 to 56% (0/76 and 14/25) and in castrated males from 16 to 75% (10/61 and 21/28), but the high incidence (96-98%) and short latent period of tumour induction were not altered in intact females. In ovariectomized females the tumour incidence was not altered by Ovulen (82% as compared to 77%), but the latent period was reduced in both ovariectomized females and castrated males (Rudali, 1974).

Heston et al. (1973) confirmed the production of chromophobe adenomas of the hypophysis in C57BL females given 20 µg Enovid/g of food for lifespan (36/49 compared to 15/51 in controls). In BALB/c females treated similarly, an increased incidence of non-metastasizing epithelial tumorous lesions of the cervix and vagina was reported in excess over controls. The incidence of ovarian tumours was not increased in treated C3H and C_3HfB females, and the incidence of mammary tumours was decreased in treated C3H females.

Twenty female BALB/c mice were fed a liquid diet (Metrecal) containing an estimated dose of 10-12.5 µg Enovid/mouse/day for an average period of 15 months. Among 16 mice which survived 10 months or more, 3 developed pre-cancerous lesions and 2, squamous-cell carcinomas of the cervix and/or vagina. In addition, in a group of 40 mice treated with Enovid and intra-vaginal inoculations of herpesvirus type 2, 31 mice survived 10 months or more; of these, 1 developed a pre-cancerous lesion and 6, squamous-cell carcinomas of the cervix and/or vagina. In 15/20 control mice which survived 10 months or more, 1 pre-cancerous lesion of the cervix was detected (Muñoz, 1973).

Mestranol administered alone in the diet at an estimated daily intake of 0.25 µg/mouse/day increased the incidence of breast tumours to 85% in castrated male RIII mice within 8 months compared with an incidence of 42% in intact male RIII mice within 14 months. In castrated male (C3H x RIII)F_1 mice fed 2.5 µg/mouse/day, 95% developed breast tumours within 28 weeks compared with 15% of controls within 69 weeks. No effects on the latency or on the high spontaneous mammary tumour incidence were observed in females (Rudali et al., 1971).

Rudali et al. (1972) studied the effects of mestranol on the induction of breast tumours in castrated male (C3H x RIII)F_1 mice. Administration of mestranol in the diet at an estimated intake of 75 µg/kg bw/day resulted in an increased incidence of mammary tumours (26/32), with an average latent period of 30 weeks, as compared with an incidence of 10/61 at 82 weeks in untreated control castrates.

The Committee on Safety of Medicines (1972) coordinated a trial of mestranol alone or in combination with several progestins (norethynodrel, ethynodiol diacetate, norethisterone, chlormadinone acetate and lynestrenol). The drugs were evaluated for carcinogenicity by incorporation into the diet of 2 strains of mice (CF-LP and Swiss) for 80 weeks. The doses were identified only as low (2-5 times the human dose), medium (50-150 times) and high (200-400 times). The amounts administered were not specified.

Mestranol alone increased the incidence of pituitary tumours in 120 male and 120 female treated CF-LP mice (12 and 17, respectively, compared with 2 and 6 in male and female controls). Larger increases were found in both males and females given the combinations with progestins, incidences ranging from 15-47 in males and from 27-42 in females per group of 120 animals.

In groups of 47-123 Swiss mice administered mestranol alone or in combination with lynestrenol, malignant mammary tumours were found in about 4% of both males and females given mestranol alone compared with 0% in controls. In combination with lynestrenol, the incidence in females increased to 6%, but no such tumours occurred in males.

Rat: In a group of 21 female Wistar rats given daily gastric instillations of 3 mg Enovid 6 times per week for 50 weeks, no breast tumours were observed, compared with 1/54 in a group of untreated controls. In a further group of 47 female rats given a similar dose of Enovid together with 2-5 mg 3-methylcholanthrene 6 times per week for 52 weeks, the incidence of mammary tumours was neither increased not decreased when compared

with that produced by the administration of 3-methylcholanthrene alone
(Gruenstein et al., 1964). Some inhibition of the induction of mammary
tumours following a single dose of 15 or 20 mg 7,12-dimethylbenzanthracene
(DMBA) was observed after Enovid administration (Weisburger et al., 1968;
Stern & Mickey, 1969).

The Committee on Safety of Medicines (1972) (see under "mouse" for
details) reported an increase in the incidence of malignant mammary tumours
in female rats given mestranol alone for 104 weeks. The incidence was 5%
in 50 controls compared with 22% in 100 treated animals. Mestranol alone
was not tested in males. In combination with progestins (norethynodrel
and norethisterone) the incidence of malignant mammary tumours in males
(12-20% compared with 0% in controls) and females (6-30% compared with 5-7%
in controls) was significantly increased. In male rats, the incidences of
benign liver-cell tumours were 2.5 and 4.0% in groups of 120 and 40 controls
compared with 8-29% in groups of 120 rats administered norethynodrel plus
mestranol and 12-23% in groups of 120 rats administered norethisterone plus
mestranol.

Dog: In a preliminary report, mestranol alone or in combination with
one of three progestins (ethynerone, Wy-4355 or anagestone acetate) was
given daily for 3 of every 4 weeks to groups of 16 female beagle dogs at
doses 2, 10 and 25 times the human dose for 42-56 months. It is reported
that mammary nodules (ranging from cystic lobular hyperplasia to adenocarcinomas) were seen in dogs given the progestin/mestranol mixture, but
not in dogs given mestranol alone. Exact details of tumour incidences are
not reported (Wazeter et al., 1973).

Monkey: In a study still in progress at the time of reporting, an
adenocarcinoma of the mammary gland was observed after 18 months in 1/6
female rhesus monkeys following administration of 1 mg Enovid per day.
There were widespread metastases associated with the tumour (Kirschstein
et al., 1972). {Assessment of this result is made difficult by the fact
that the animals were 6-8 years old at the beginning of treatment and had
borne at least one infant. However, the incidence of spontaneous breast
cancer in the colony was reported to be very low.}

In a further study still in progress, mestranol alone or in combination with one of three progestins (ethynerone, Wy-4355 or anagestone acetate), when administered to groups of 16 female monkeys at dose levels in the order of 2, 10 and 50 times the human dose, produced no tumours within 42-56 months (Wazeter et al., 1973).

(b) Subcutaneous and/or intramuscular injection

Rat: Repeated s.c. injection of 10 or 100 µg Enovid/day into 2 groups of 25 female Sprague-Dawley rats for 40 days reduced the number of mammary tumours/rat produced by a single i.v. injection of 5 mg DMBA given on day 25 of treatment. The average number of tumours/rat was 10.9 in 37 controls given DMBA alone compared with 7.6 and 3.9 in rats given 10 or 100 µg Enovid/day, respectively (Welsch & Meites, 1969).

3.2 Other relevant biological data

See section, "General Remarks on the Sex Hormones", and pp. 38-40.

3.3 Observations in man

See section, "Oestrogens and Progestins in Relation to Human Cancer", p. 219.

4. Comments on Data Reported and Evaluation[1]

4.1 Animal data

Mestranol was tested in mice and rats by the oral route; in most studies it was administered in combination with progestins. When administered alone, the incidences of pituitary tumours were increased in both sexes of one strain of mice, and malignant mammary tumours were produced in males and females of another strain. It also produced an increased incidence of mammary tumours in castrated male mice and of malignant mammary tumours in female rats.

---

[1] This section should be read in conjunction with the section, "General Conclusions on Hormones", p. 235.

In experiments where mestranol was administered to female mice in combination with norethynodrel (as Enovid), pituitary, mammary, vaginal and cervical tumours were produced. In rats, combinations with norethynodrel and norethisterone produced an excess of benign liver-cell tumours in male rats and increased the incidence of malignant mammary tumours in rats of both sexes.

The results in dogs and monkeys were difficult to assess since the studies were still in progress at the time of reporting.

4.2 Human data

No case reports or epidemiological studies on the effects of mestranol alone were available to the Working Group. Epidemiological studies on steroid hormones in oestrogen-progestin contraceptive preparations have been summarized in the section "Oestrogens and Progestins in Relation to Human Cancer", p. 223.

5. References

Blacow, N.W., ed. (1972) *Martindale. The Extra Pharmacopoeia*, 26th ed., London, The Pharmaceutical Press, p. 1661

Committee on Safety of Medicines (1972) *Carcinogenicity tests of oral contraceptives*, London, HMSO

Dunn, T.B. (1969) Cancer of the uterine cervix in mice fed a liquid diet containing an antifertility drug. *J. nat. Cancer Inst.*, 43, 671-692

Gruenstein, M., Shay, H. & Shimkin, M.B. (1964) Lack of effect of norethynodrel (Enovid) on methylcholanthrene-induced mammary carcinogenesis in female rats. *Cancer Res.*, 24, 1656-1658

Heston, W.E., Vlahakis, G. & Desmukes, B. (1973) Effects of the antifertility drug Enovid in five strains of mice with particular regard to carcinogenesis. *J. nat. Cancer Inst.*, 51, 209-224

Kastrup, E.K., ed. (1973) *Facts and Comparisons*, St. Louis, Missouri, Facts & Comparisons Inc.

Kirschstein, R.L., Rabson, A.S. & Rusten, G.W. (1972) Infiltrating duct carcinoma of the mammary gland of a rhesus monkey after administration of an oral contraceptive: A preliminary report. *J. nat. Cancer Inst.*, 48, 551-556

Muñoz, N. (1973) Effect of herpesvirus type 2 and hormonal imbalance on the uterine cervix of the mouse. *Cancer Res.*, 33, 1504-1508

Poel, W.E. (1966) Pituitary tumors in mice after prolonged feeding of synthetic progestins. *Science*, 154, 402-403

Rudali, G. (1974) Induction of tumors in mice with synthetic sex hormones. *Gann Monograph* (in press)

Rudali, G., Coezy, E., Frederic, F. & Apiou, F. (1971) Susceptibility of mice of different strains to the mammary carcinogenic action of natural and synthetic oestrogens. *Rev. europ. Etudes Clin. Biol.*, 16, 425-429

Rudali, G., Coezy, E. & Chemama, R. (1972) Mammary carcinogenesis in female and male mice receiving contraceptives or gestagens. *J. nat. Cancer Inst.*, 49, 813-819

Stern, E. & Mickey, M.R. (1969) Effects of a cyclic steroid contraceptive regimen on mammary gland tumor induction in rats. *Brit. J. Cancer*, 23, 391-400

Wazeter, F.X., Geil, R.G., Berliner, V.R. & Lamar, J.K. (1973) Studies of tumorigenic and diabetogenic potential of certain oral contraceptive steroids in female dogs and monkeys. Toxicol. appl. Pharmacol., 25, 498

Weisburger, J.H., Weisburger, E.K., Griswold, D.P., Jr & Casey, A.E. (1968) Reduction of carcinogen-induced breast cancer in rats by an antifertility drug. Life Sci., 7, 259-266

Welsch, C.W. & Meites, J. (1969) Effects of norethynodrel-mestranol combination (Enovid) on development and growth of carcinogen-induced mammary tumors in female rats. Cancer, 23, 601-607

OESTRADIOL-17β

1. Chemical and Physical Data

1.1 Synonyms and trade names*

Chem. Abstr. No.: 50-28-2

Dihydrofollicular hormone; dihydrofolliculin; dihydrotheelin; 3,17β-dihydroxyestra-1,3,5-triene; 3,17β-dihydroxyoestra-1,3,5-triene; 3,17β-dihydroxy-1,3,5(10)-estratriene; 3,17β-dihydroxy-1,3,5(10)-oestratriene; dihydroxyestrin; dihydroxyoestrin; 3,17-epidihydroxyestratriene; 3,17-epidihydroxyoestratriene; estradiol; oestradiol; estradiol-17β; β-estradiol (formerly called α-estradiol); β-oestradiol (formerly called α-oestradiol); cis-estradiol; cis-oestradiol; d-estradiol; d-oestradiol; d-3,17β-estradiol; d-3,17β-oestradiol; D-3,17β-estradiol; D-3,17β-oestradiol; 17β-estradiol; 17β-oestradiol; estra-1,3,5(10)-triene-3,17β-diol; oestra-1,3,5(10)-triene-3,17β-diol; 1,3,5-estratriene-3,17β-diol; 1,3,5-oestratriene-3,17β-diol; 17β-OH-estradiol; 17β-OH-oestradiol; (17β)-estra-1,3,5(10)-triene-3,17-diol; (17β)-oestra-1,3,5(10)-triene-3,17-diol; 1,3,5(10)-estratriene-3,17β-diol; 1,3,5(10)-oestratriene-3,17β-diol

Ablacton; Altrad; Androtardyl-Oestr.; Aquadiol; Bardiol; Benzo-gynoestryl; Benzo-Gynoestryl 5; Ciclo Complex; Climastat; Clivion; Combidurin; Depofemin; Dihydromenformon; Dimenformon; Dimenformon Prolong.; Diogyn; Diogynets; Duogynon; Emmenovis; Emonovister; Estradurin; Estradurine; Estraldine; Estrandron; Estrandron Prolong.; Estrovite; Femestral; Femogen; Folicular; Folicular Depot; Foliteston Retard; Gravibinan; Gravibinon; Ginosedol; Gynecormone; Gynergon; Gynoestrel; Gynoestryl; Heptylate de Test.; Hormonin; Lamdiol; Luteo Folicular; Lutestron; Lutestron Dep.; Lut Ovociclina; Lutrogen; Macrodiol; Nordicol; Oestergon; Oestradiol R; Oestro-glandol; Oestrogynal; Ovahormon; Ova Repos; Ovasterol; Ovastevol;

---

* Trade names include mixtures containing oestradiol-17β

Ovestin; Ovex; Ovex Prolong.; Ovociclina; Ovocyclin; Ovocycline; Ovocylin; Ovolacer; Primodian D; Primodian Depot; Primofol; Primogyn Depot; Primosiston; Profoliol; Progynon; Progynon B Oleoso; Progynon D; Progynon Depot; Progynon-DH; Progynon Pomada; Progynon Retard; Progynon S; Progynova; C Progynova; Proluton-Oestradiol; Proluton Z; Stroluten; Syndiol; Test.-Oestr. R; Testo Folicular; Trioestrine; Trioestrine R; Trioestrine Vitam.

1.2 <u>Chemical formula and molecular weight</u>

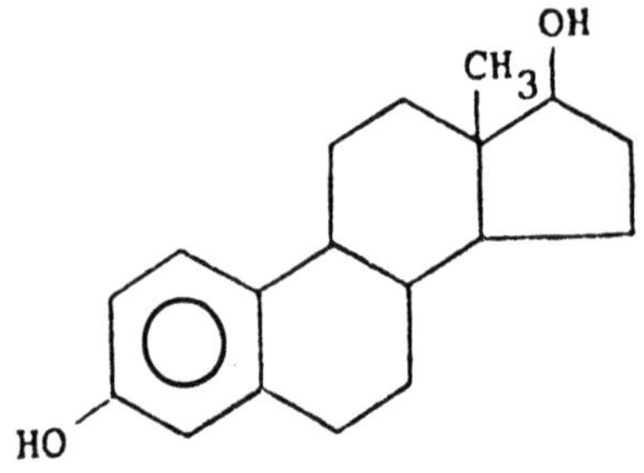

$C_{18}H_{24}O_2$

Mol. wt: 272.4

1.3 <u>Chemical and physical properties of the pure substance</u>

(<u>a</u>) <u>Description</u>: White, or creamy-white crystals (from 80% alcohol)

(<u>b</u>) <u>Melting-point</u>: 173-179°C

(<u>c</u>) <u>Absorption spectrometry</u>: λ_{max} 225 and 280 nm

(<u>d</u>) <u>Optical rotation</u>: $\{\alpha\}_D^{25}$ +76 to +83° (10% w/v in dioxane)

(<u>e</u>) <u>Solubility</u>: Almost insoluble in water; soluble at 25°C in 95% ethanol (1 in 30), acetone (1 in 17); freely soluble in chloroform, dioxane and aqueous solutions of alkali hydroxides; sparingly soluble in vegetable oils

1.4 Technical products and impurities

Oestradiol-17β is available in the United States as an aqueous injection, NF, as pellets, NF, and as tablets in combinations with oestriol and oestrone. Solutions of the following ester derivatives in vegetable oil are also available in several concentrations as injections in oil, NF:

benzoate, cypionate (cyclopentylpropionate), dipropionate and valerate. A polyoestradiol phosphate injection for treatment of prostatic carcinoma is also made (Kastrup, 1973).

2. Production, Use, Occurrence and Analysis

2.1 Production and use[1]

Isolation of oestradiol-17β was reported by MacCorquodale et al. (1936), and numerous methods of synthesis from other steroids were subsequently reported. It can be isolated from pregnant mares' urine, but the single US manufacturer is believed to synthesize it from diosgenin. It can be made by the reduction of oestrone or by degradation of diosgenin to 1-dehydrotestosterone, which is converted by pyrolysis to oestradiol-17β.

The US company which produces oestradiol-17β also produces oestradiol valerate, and another US company produces oestradiol cypionate (cyclopentylpropionate). However, no data are available on the quantity of these chemicals produced in the US.

In 1972, 60 kg of oestradiol benzoate were reported to have been imported through the principal US customs districts (US Tariff Commission, 1973), but separate data on US imports of oestradiol-17β or of its other derivatives are not available.

Oestradiol-17β and its ester derivatives are used in human medicine for the treatment of such conditions as amenorrhea, breast carcinoma, hypogenitalism, menopausal syndrome, postmenopausal osteoporosis, postpartum breast engorgement, prostatic carcinoma and senile vaginitis. In such applications, they are frequently used in combination with other hormones, e.g., androgens and other oestrogens (Kastrup, 1973). Total US sales of oestradiol-17β and its ester derivatives for use in human medicine are estimated to be less than 100 kg annually.

---

[1] Data from Chemical Information Services, Stanford Research Institute, USA

Data on production of oestradiol-17β in the countries of Western Europe are not available, but it is believed to be manufactured by at least one company in the Federal Republic of Germany and by one in France. Total sales of oestradiol-17β in hormone specialties in Western Europe in 1972 are estimated to have been less than 170 kg. Sales in the Federal Republic of Germany represented approximately 45% of the total, with lesser amounts sold in Belgium, France, Italy, The Netherlands, Spain and the United Kingdom.

Oestradiol benzoate is approved for use in the US as the principal ingredient in implants for heifers, lambs and steers for promoting growth and feed efficiency. Oestradiol monopalmitate is approved for use as an injection for roasting chickens to produce more uniform fat distribution. However, no residues of these oestradiol esters must remain in the edible, uncooked tissue of the treated animals (US Code of Federal Regulations, 1973). The quantity of oestradiol benzoate used as a growth promoter in heifers, lambs and steers may have increased dramatically in recent months as a result of the US Food and Drug Administration ban on the use of diethylstilboestrol implants as growth promoters for these animals.

The use of such oestrogenic hormones as growth promoters in animals is forbidden in some European countries; in other countries they are still used.

Oestradiol-17β is used for veterinary purposes in horses, cattle, sheep, swine and dogs in replacement therapy for underdeveloped females, in the treatment of incontinence and vaginitis of spayed bitches, in reproductive disorders and in other conditions (Merck & Co., 1968). No data are available on the quantity of oestradiol-17β and its esters consumed in the US in these ways.

2.2 Occurrence

Oestradiol-17β is a widely occurring natural oestrogen (see section, "General Remarks on the Sex Hormones", p. 30, for further information).

2.3 Analysis

General methods of analysis are summarized in the section, "General Remarks on the Sex Hormones", p. 40.

3. Biological Data Relevant to the Evaluation of Carcinogenic Risk to Man

3.1 Carcinogenicity and related studies in animals

(a) Subcutaneous and/or intramuscular injection

Mouse: Hooker & Pfeiffer (1942) induced interstitial-cell tumours of the testis in 10/24 male Strong A mice surviving s.c. injections of either 16.6 or 50 µg oestradiol benzoate in sesame oil once a week for 8 months or more. Both doses were equally effective. Administration of 1.25 mg testosterone propionate together with 50 µg oestradiol benzoate weekly reduced the incidence of testicular tumours to 2/15, and the time of induction was longer (14 months). The authors described in detail the accompanying regressive changes in the testis and emphasized that atrophy was less marked in these mice than in strains which do not develop interstitial-cell tumours with chronic oestrogen exposure (c.f., Bonser & Robson, 1940).

Gardner (1941) reported the effects of weekly s.c. injections of 16.6 or 50 µg oestradiol benzoate on the incidence of pituitary and mammary tumours in hybrid mice derived from reciprocal matings of the C57 strain, which has a high incidence of oestrogen-induced pituitary tumours (Gardner & Strong, 1940) but no susceptibility to breast tumour induction, and CBA mice, which do not develop pituitary tumours with oestrogen but which have a high spontaneous incidence of mammary cancer. Treatment of groups of 20-30 mice was started when the animals were 4-8 weeks old and was continued for lifespan. When the mother was from the high pituitary tumour incidence strain (C57), such tumours were found in 53% of hybrid females and in 83% of the males. When the mother was from the CBA strain, the corresponding incidences of pituitary tumours were 32% and 75%. Mammary tumours (58% in males and 60% in females) occurred only in hybrid mice with a CBA mother and were presumed to be dependent on the presence of the mammary tumour virus (MTV). The percentage of lymphoid tumours in treated groups (9-17%) was higher than in control groups, but the differences were not statistically significant.

Bonser & Robson (1940) found mammary carcinomas after 20-40 weeks of treatment in 9/31 male RIII mice given weekly s.c. injections of 50 µg oestradiol dipropionate, but 18 of the initial 31 treated mice had died by the 20th week of the experiment. In untreated RIII strain mice the incidence of breast cancer in females living more than 7 months (breeding status not given) was about 63%. No breast tumours occurred in males of the CBA strain injected with the same dose of oestradiol dipropionate; however, no spontaneous mammary tumours had ever been observed in the CBA strain maintained by these workers, presumably because they lacked the MTV, in contrast to the related line reported by Gardner (1941).

Free oestradiol-17β injected s.c. in sesame oil at a dose of 80 µg twice weekly for 6 months (total dose, 3.3-4.2 mg) was found to be toxic (Bischoff et al., 1942a), and the treatment did not increase the incidence of breast tumours in groups of 40 intact or 40 ovariectomized female Marsh-Buffalo mice above that found in untreated controls. However, lymphosarcomas occurred earlier (between 3 and 6 months) and in a higher incidence (28% in intact, 47% in ovariectomized) than in the controls, in which 10% had tumours, the first tumour appearing at 12 months. Similar results were obtained with discontinuous treatment in groups of 36-43 intact and castrated males of the same strain (Bischoff et al., 1942b). A total dose of 3.5 mg oestradiol-17β was injected on 195 out of 360 days, with interruptions of treatment due to toxicity. Lymphoid tumours occurred in 34% of castrates, compared with 8% in intact treated males and 5% in controls. The tumours in castrates developed much earlier (at 6-14 months) than in the other groups.

The effects of s.c. administration of oestrogens on lymphoid tumour development in large numbers of seven different mouse strains have been detailed (Gardner et al., 1944), but unfortunately the nature of the oestrogen used in particular experiments is not clearly defined. Oestradiol-17β was rather more effective than were the other compounds tested. In one series, oestradiol dipropionate given s.c. in sesame oil once a week for 10 weeks increased the incidence of lymphoid tumours in C3H mice (sex not stated) by 16.7% with 10 µg doses, by 22% with 25 µg and by 23% with 50 µg. The incidence of tumours in untreated mice was low (total, 1.3%) in all strains tested.

Kirschbaum et al. (1953) found that mice of the BALB/c and CBA strains less than 57 weeks old were relatively resistant to the induction of lymphoid tumours by either X-rays, methylcholanthrene or oestradiol dipropionate (5 µg in oil s.c. weekly for 14 weeks), but that in the BALB/c mice the combination of oestradiol dipropionate with 200 rad whole body irradiation increased the incidence from 3/47 to 16/71. Although 400 rad alone were no more effective than were 200 rad, the incidence of lymphomas was greater (12/30 by 43 weeks of age in BALB/c mice and 15/27 by 57 weeks in CBA mice) when 400 rad was combined with 5 µg oestradiol dipropionate given weekly for 14 weeks. Thymectomy abolished the synergistic action of these two agents. The leukaemogenic action of methylcholanthrene was not increased by combination with oestradiol-17β. In DBA mice, however, the same dose of oestradiol dipropionate increased the leukaemogenic activity of both X-rays and methylcholanthrene, although the oestrogen itself was not a significant inducer of lymphoid tumours.

Invasive cervical lesions or carcinomas occurred in 4/10 female hybrid mice (C3H x PM strain) administered 16.6 µg oestradiol benzoate s.c., once weekly, starting at 4-9 weeks of age. In 25 female mice of the reciprocal hybrid (PM x C3H) strain receiving 16.6 or 25 µg oestradiol benzoate s.c., carcinomas or evasive epithelial lesions arose from the uterine cervix in 8 mice and from the vagina in 1 mouse after 29 weeks or more of treatment. No uterine, cervical or vaginal carcinomas were found in 82 controls (Pan & Gardner, 1948).

Four female mice of the BC strain and one female CBA mouse, which were injected s.c. with 16.6 µg oestradiol dipropionate in sesame oil once weekly commencing at ages ranging from 41-65 weeks, had tumours of the uterus at 78-89 weeks. Two of the BC strain also had cervical tumours (Gardner & Ferrigno, 1956). {The total incidence of these lesions in the treated mice cannot be assessed from the data nor is the incidence of similar lesions in untreated mice known.}

In an unspecified number of female mice of reciprocal crosses between the C57 and CBA strains injected s.c. with weekly doses of 16.6 or 50 µg oestradiol benzoate (vehicle not stated) commencing at 4-8 weeks of age, cervical lesions ranging from invasion to gross tumours which invaded adjacent tissues were seen in 15/24 (62%) of mice with C57 mothers and in 10/20 (50%) with CBA mothers and surviving for more than 52 weeks. In the latter group there was a high incidence of mammary cancer, which reduced the lifespan. No lesions were seen before 59 weeks in either group. Of 10 mice in the two groups which survived more than 86 weeks, 4 had no lesions at death. Although none of the tumours metastasized, it was concluded that the range of lesions seen probably represented various stages of carcinoma development. No cervical tumours occurred among an equal number of control mice (Allen & Gardner, 1941). {Support for the probability of the malignant nature of these cervical lesions comes from an earlier observation (Gardner et al., 1938) that an advanced carcinoma of the cervix which had metastasized to lymph nodes was found in a C3H mouse which received a total of 1.05 mg oestradiol benzoate between 6 and 51 weeks of age. The tumour was transplanted successfully into untreated mice of both sexes.}

Newborn mouse: Takasugi & Bern (1964) found that female mice of 4 strains receiving 5 µg oestradiol-17β daily for the first 5 days after birth showed hyperplastic and epidermoid vaginal lesions at 32-63 weeks of age: 16/23 in A/Crgl strain, 6/14 in BALB/cCrgl, 4/16 in C57BL/Crgl and 3/15 in RIII/Crgl. No lesions were found in 6 oestrogenized C3H/Crgl mice at 44 weeks of age, and one lesion occurred in 1/5 C57BL/Crgl controls, although most of these mice showed persistent vaginal cornification. Vaginal concretions ("stones") were found in almost all mice showing vaginal lesions, but their role has yet to be assessed. {These results parallel those found by Dunn & Green (1963) after neonatal diethylstilboestrol administration to mice and should be considered in the light of clinical findings of vaginal cancer in the daughters of diethylstilboestrol-treated mothers (see p. 66).}

Kimura & Nandi (1967) injected female mice of the BALB/cCrgl strain with 25, 5 or 0.1 µg oestradiol-17β as an aqueous suspension daily for the first 5 days of life. Approximately half the animals in each group were ovariectomized at 16-17 weeks of age. All mice receiving the two larger doses and 88% of mice receiving the smaller dose of oestradiol-17β developed persistent vaginal cornification. This cornification was maintained after ovariectomy in all mice which had received 25 or 5 µg oestradiol-17β but not in those which had received 0.1 µg. The mice were killed between 64 and 73 weeks of age, and vaginal epithelial downgrowths were found in 100% of 16 and 11 intact mice which had been given 25 or 5 µg and in 84% of 19 intact mice which had received 0.1 µg. In the corresponding ovariectomized groups, the incidences of downgrowths were reduced to 94, 50 and 0% of 16, 10 and 9 mice, respectively. Hyperplastic vaginal lesions resembling epidermoid carcinoma were found at termination in 19/27 intact mice and in 8/26 ovariectomized mice given 25 or 5 µg oestradiol, but in only 3/19 intact mice and 0/9 ovariectomized mice which had been given 0.1 µg. The mean ovarian weights of all the oestradiol-17β-treated intact mice were more than twice those of the controls. Epithelial downgrowth was found in the vaginas of 5/10 intact controls, but no hyperplastic lesions were seen. Four ovariectomized controls had no vaginal dysplasias.

Data on neonatally oestrogenized female mouse vagina have been summarized by Takasugi et al. (1970). Evidence for the neonatal "selection" by oestrogen of a special cell population in the vagina and uterine cervix in mice, which later gives rise to abnormal lesions, has been presented by Forsberg (1972, 1973) and by Takasugi & Kamishima (1973). Increased mammary tumorigenesis in MTV-bearing mice after neonatal oestradiol-17β treatment has been reported (Mori, 1968a,b; Bern et al., 1973); and metaplastic lesions have also been found to occur in various sex accessories, including prostatic lobes, in neonatally oestrogenized male C3H/MS mice (Mori, 1967).

Guinea-pig: Lipschütz & Iglesias (1938) described the induction of uterine and extra-uterine tumours by the injection of oestrogens into ovariectomized female guinea-pigs. In 22/24 guinea-pigs given s.c. injections three times weekly of 20-80 µg oestradiol benzoate in olive oil (Progynon B), multiple tumours arose in the uterus, in the ventral surface of the stomach, in the spleen, in the mesentery, in the surface of the diaphragm and in other abdominal locations after 2-4 months. Tumours never occurred in the thorax, nor with the vehicle alone. The unesterified oestrogens were less active than was the benzoate (Lipschütz & Vargas, 1939a).

Intact and castrated male guinea-pigs were susceptible to tumour induction by 80 μg oestradiol benzoate given three times weekly, but the size and extent of the abdominal lesions were less (Koref et al., 1939). The tumours regressed after cessation of the treatment (Lipschütz et al., 1939). The structure and origin of these tumours has been described and their significance discussed by Lipschütz & Vargas (1941): histologically they have varying degrees of fibromyomatous and fibromatous proliferation, with some suggestion of transition to sarcoma. The tentative conclusion is that they are benign lesions peculiar to the oestrogen-treated guinea-pig.

(b) Subcutaneous implantation (pellets)

Mouse: When castrated male (C3H x RIII)F_1 mice (carrying the MTV) were given a s.c. implant of a pellet containing 0.5-1 mg oestradiol-17β in paraffin wax at the age of 10 or 70 days, 15/16 (94%) and 18/18 (100%), respectively, developed mammary cancer. Such tumours occurred in 17% of castrated controls the mean latency period being 69 weeks, compared with 25-27 weeks in treated mice. In C3H and RIII strains the incidences of mammary cancer found in groups of castrated males treated at 10 days of age with oestradiol-17β paraffin pellets were 72 and 82%, respectively. Mammary tumours occurred in only 16% of males of the NLC strain and in 0% of C57BL males given similar implants (Rudali et al., 1971).

Lymphoid tumours, almost all thymic lymphosarcomas, arose in 27/84 male BALB/c mice before 57 weeks of age after the s.c. implantation of a 1-2 mg pellet of oestradiol dipropionate. No lymphosarcomas were observed in 240 control mice. Females of this strain did not survive the treatment for a significant period (Kirschbaum et al., 1953).

Of 20 BALB/c female mice treated every 3-4 months with 5 mg implants of an oestradiol-17β-cholesterol mixture for an average period of 15 months, 17 mice survived 10 months or more and 2 developed precancerous lesions and 5 developed squamous-cell carcinomas of the cervix and/or of the vagina. Of 40 mice treated with s.c. pellets of oestradiol-17β and intravaginal inoculations of herpesvirus type 2, 36 mice survived 10 months or more and 10 developed precancerous lesions and 7 developed squamous-cell carcinomas of the cervix and/or of the vagina. In 15/20 control mice which survived 10 months or more, no cervical or vaginal lesions were found (Muñoz, 1973).

Rat: Rats from the Wistar Albino (Glaxo) strain (WAG), albino rats of the Royal Cancer Hospital (London) strain and hooded rats originally derived from the MRC (London) strain were given two pellets of 5-6 mg oestradiol-17β or oestradiol dipropionate, the initial implant at the age of 4 weeks and a further implant after 1-3 months (Mackenzie, 1955). Pituitary enlargement due to chromophobe adenomas (320 mg; range, 29-606 mg) was common in all strains, occurring in 69/92 rats. Mammary cancers developed in 10/27 female WAG rats between 29 and 64 weeks of age; no such tumours were seen in 5 males which survived for longer than 64 weeks. Mammary cancers occurred in 2/38 female Cancer Hospital rats and in 6/19 female rats of the hooded MRC strain which lived longer than 29 weeks. No carcinomas of the breast occurred among equivalent numbers (not stated) of breeding or control rats of the strains used.

Gillman & Gilbert (1955) induced pituitary tumours in adult Wistar albino rats (sex not stated) by implantation of pellets of oestradiol benzoate weighing 6-8 mg. The incidence of tumours is not clear from the data given, but an average pituitary weight of 217 mg was recorded in 8 rats at 14-21 weeks after the start of the experiment; and this average was maintained or increased up to 50 weeks in 73 other rats. Weekly injections of 20 µg thyroxine accelerated pituitary hypertrophy in a smaller group treated with oestradiol benzoate pellets. The treatment with oestradiol-17β did not induce pituitary hypertrophy in groups of rats fed a diet containing 0.5% thiouracil.

Hamster: In an extensive review of the induction of malignant renal tumours (not specified) in hamsters, Kirkman (1959) reported the occurrence of these tumours in 15/15 intact and in 12/12 castrated males and in 10/16 ovariectomized females given one or more sub-pannicular 20 mg pellets of oestradiol-17β every 21 weeks. The age at autopsy varied between 45 and 81 weeks for males and between 24 and 58 weeks for the ovariectomized females. No kidney tumours were found in 6 treated intact females, nor among intact or castrated controls of either sex.

Guinea-pig: Lipschütz & Vargas (1939b) reported the appearance of fibromyomas in the uterus, mesentery and other abdominal sites in female guinea-pigs ovariectomized 3 months before the s.c. implantation of a 20 or 50 mg pellet of oestradiol-17β. Fibromyomas were detected as early as 19 days after the start of treatment and occurred in all animals. The pellets lost up to 10 mg in weight over 7 weeks of the experiment. Similar results were obtained by Woodruff (1941) with oestradiol benzoate, and by Riesco (1947) with oestradiol dipropionate. {For the nature of these tumours see studies reported under "Subcutaneous and/or intramuscular injection".}

Monkey: Engle et al. (1943) observed the effects of total doses of 600-825 mg oestradiol-17β implanted s.c. at intervals of 5-6 weeks over a 24-28 month period in 5 female rhesus monkeys. Cystic hyperplasia of the breast occurred, but no tumours were found.

Five Capuchin monkeys (Cebus apella) were given s.c. implants of oestradiol dipropionate and/or oestradiol-17β. In some cases the pellet consisted of the pure oestrogen and in others of a mixture of 40% oestrogen and 60% cholesterol. The amount of oestrogen absorbed per day was about 250-700 μg/animal, and the total duration of treatment ranged from 29-145 weeks. In addition, 3 animals received s.c. injections of other oestradiol esters (100-200 μg) twice weekly. A high degree of cystic and polypous glandular hyperplasia of the uterine mucosa developed in all animals. The only tumour observed was found in the longest survivor and was an adenocarcinoma or endothelioma of the pericardium, but it was considered not to be due to the treatment (Iglesias & Lipschütz, 1947).

3.2 Other relevant biological data

See section, "General Remarks on the Sex Hormones", and pp. 38-40.

3.3 Observations in man

See section, "Oestrogens and Progestins in Relation to Human Cancer", p. 219.

4. Comments on Data Reported and Evaluation[1]

4.1 Animal Data

Oestradiol-17β was tested in mice, rats, hamsters and guinea-pigs by subcutaneous injection or implantation. Its administration resulted in an increased incidence of mammary, pituitary, uterine, cervical, vaginal and lymphoid tumours and interstitial-cell tumours of the testis in mice. In rats, there was an increased incidence of mammary and pituitary tumours. In hamsters, malignant kidney tumours occurred with a high incidence in intact or castrated males and in ovariectomized but not in intact females. In guinea-pigs, diffuse fibromyomatous abdominal lesions of uncertain histological interpretation were observed. Subcutaneous injections in neonatal mice resulted in precancerous and cancerous vaginal lesions in later life.

The studies in monkeys could not be assessed since they were limited in group size and duration.

Oestradiol-17β treatment increased the incidence of mammary and pituitary tumours in strains of mice having a spontaneous incidence of these tumours. The spontaneous occurrence can be related either to the presence of a virus or to a particular genetic susceptibility. No evidence of the possible role of a virus has been ascertained for rats.

The role of the hormonal balance in the development and persistence of these tumours and possible synergisms with other carcinogenic factors in increasing the incidence of lymphoid tumours has been discussed (see section, "General Remarks on the Sex Hormones", p. 27).

4.2 Human data

No case reports or epidemiological studies were available to the Working Group. Epidemiological studies on steroid hormones used in oestrogen treatment have been summarized in the section, "Oestrogens and Progestins in Relation to Human Cancer", p. 219.

---

[1] This section should also be read in conjunction with the section, "General Conclusions on Hormones", p. 235.

5. References

Allen, E. & Gardner, W.U. (1941) Cancer of the cervix of the uterus in hybrid mice following long-continued administration of estrogen. Cancer Res., 1, 359-366

Bern, H.A., Mori, T. & Young, P.N. (1973) Preliminary report on the effects of perinatal exposure to hormones on the mammary gland of female BALB/cf.C3H mice. In: Proceedings of the 8th Meeting on Mammary Cancer in Experimental Animals and Man, Airlie House, Virginia, p. 12

Bischoff, F., Long, M.L., Rupp, J.J. & Clarke, G.J. (1942a) Carcinogenic effect of estradiol and of theelin in Marsh-Buffalo mice. Cancer Res., 2, 52-55

Bischoff, F., Long, M.L., Rupp, J.J. & Clarke, G.J. (1942b) Influence of toxic amounts of estrin upon intact and castrated male Marsh-Buffalo mice. Cancer Res., 2, 198-199

Bonser, G.M. & Robson, J.M. (1940) The effects of prolonged oestrogen administration upon male mice of various strains: development of testicular tumours in the Strong A strain. J. Path. Bact., 51, 9-22

Dunn, T.B. & Green, A.W. (1963) Cysts of the epididymis, cancer of the cervix, granular cell myoblastoma and other lesions after estrogen injection in newborn mice. J. nat. Cancer Inst., 31, 425-438

Engle, E.T., Krakower, C. & Haagensen, C.D. (1943) Estrogen administration to aged female monkeys with no resultant tumors. Cancer Res., 3, 858-866

Forsberg, J.-G. (1972) Estrogen, vaginal cancer and vaginal development. Amer. J. Obstet. Gynec., 113, 83-87

Forsberg, J.-G. (1973) Cervicovaginal epithelium: its origin and development. Amer. J. Obstet. Gynec., 115, 1025-1043

Gardner, W.U. (1941) The effect of estrogen on the incidence of mammary and pituitary tumors in hybrid mice. Cancer Res., 1, 345-358

Gardner, W.U. & Ferrigno, M. (1956) Unusual neoplastic lesions of the uterine horns of estrogen-treated mice. J. nat. Cancer Inst., 17, 601-613

Gardner, W.U. & Strong, L.C. (1940) Strain-limited development of tumors of the pituitary gland in mice receiving estrogens. Yale J. Biol. Med., 12, 543-549

Gardner, W.U., Allen, E., Smith, G.M. & Strong, L.C. (1938) Carcinoma of the cervix of mice receiving estrogens. J. Amer. med. Ass., 110, 1182-1183

Gardner, W.U., Dougherty, T.F. & Williams, W.L. (1944) Lymphoid tumors in mice receiving steroid hormones. Cancer Res., 4, 73-87

Gillman, J. & Gilbert, C. (1955) Modulating action of the thyroid on oestrogen-induced pituitary tumours in rats. Nature (Lond.), 175, 724-725

Hooker, C.W. & Pfeiffer, C.A. (1942) The morphology and development of testicular tumors in mice of the A strain receiving estrogens. Cancer Res., 2, 759-769

Iglesias, R. & Lipschütz, A. (1947) Effects of prolonged oestrogen administration in female New World monkeys, with observations on a pericardial neoplasm. J. Endocr., 5, 88-98

Kastrup, E.K., ed. (1973) Facts and Comparisons, St. Louis, Missouri, Facts & Comparisons Inc.

Kimura, T. & Nandi, S. (1967) Nature of induced persistent vaginal cornification in mice. IV. Changes in the vaginal epithelium of old mice treated neonatally with estradiol or testosterone. J. nat. Cancer Inst., 39, 75-83

Kirkman, H. (1959) Estrogen-induced tumors of the kidney. IV. Incidence in female Syrian hamsters. J. nat. Cancer Inst. Monogr., 1, 59-75

Kirschbaum, A., Shapiro, J.R. & Mixer, H.W. (1953) Synergistic action of leukemogenic agents. Cancer Res., 13, 262-268

Koref, O., Lipschütz, A. & Vargas, L., Jr (1939) Spécificité sexuelle et tumorigenèse. C.R. Soc. Biol. (Paris), 130, 303-306

Lipschütz, A. & Iglesias, R. (1938) Multiples tumeurs utérines et extragénitales provoquées par le benzoate d'oestradiol. C.R. Soc. Biol. (Paris), 129, 519-524

Lipschütz, A. & Vargas, L., Jr (1939a) Etude comparative sur l'action tumorigène de différentes substances oestrogènes. C.R. Soc. Biol. (Paris), 130, 9-11

Lipschütz, A. & Vargas, L., Jr (1939b) Experimental tumorigenesis with subcutaneous tablets of oestradiol. Lancet, i, 1313-1318

Lipschütz, A. & Vargas, L., Jr (1941) Structure and origin of uterine and extragenital fibroids induced experimentally in the guinea-pig by prolonged administration of estrogens. Cancer Res., 1, 236-248

Lipschütz, A., Iglesias, R. & Vargas, L., Jr (1939) Régression du fibromyome expérimental et résistance des formations tumorales épithéliales dans la carence hormonale folliculaire. C.R. Soc. Biol. (Paris), 130, 1536-1540

MacCorquodale, D.W., Thayer, S.A. & Doisy, E.A. (1936) The isolation of the principal estrogenic substance of liquor folliculi. J. biol. Chem., 115, 435-448

Mackenzie, I. (1955) The production of mammary cancer in rats using oestrogens. Brit. J. Cancer, 9, 284-299

Merck & Co. (1968) The Merck Index, 8th ed., Rahway, N.J., p. 423

Mori, T. (1967) Effects of early postnatal injections of estrogen on endocrine organs and sex accessories in male C3H/MS mice. J. Fac. Sci. Univ. Tokyo, Sect. IV, 11, 243-254

Mori, T. (1968a) Changes in reproductive organs and some other glands in old C3H/MS mice treated neonatally with low doses of estrogen. Annot. Zool. Japon., 41, 43-52

Mori, T. (1968b) Changes in the reproductive and some other organs in old C3H/MS mice given high-dose estrogen injections during neonatal life. Annot. Zool. Japon., 41, 85-94

Muñoz, N. (1973) Effect of herpesvirus type 2 and hormonal imbalance on the uterine cervix of the mouse. Cancer Res., 33, 1504-1508

Pan, S.C. & Gardner, W.U. (1948) Carcinomas of the uterine cervix and vagina in estrogen- and androgen-treated hybrid mice. Cancer Res., 8, 337-341

Riesco, A. (1947) On the bearing of time on the neoplastic action of small quantities of α-oestradiol in the endometrium of guinea-pigs. Brit. J. Cancer, 1, 166-172

Rudali, G., Coezy, E., Frederic, F. & Apiou, F. (1971) Susceptibility of mice of different strains to the mammary carcinogenic action of natural and synthetic oestrogens. Rev. europ. Et. clin. biol., 16, 425-429

Takasugi, N. & Bern, H.A. (1964) Tissue changes in mice with persistent vaginal cornification induced in early post-natal treatment with estrogen. J. nat. Cancer Inst., 33, 855-865

Takasugi, N. & Kamishima, Y. (1973) Development of vaginal epithelium showing irreversible proliferation and cornification in neonatally estrogenized mice: an electron microscope study. Develop. Growth Different., 15, 127-140

Takasugi, N., Kimura, T. & Mori, T. (1970) Irreversible changes in mouse vaginal epithelium induced by early post-natal treatment with steroid hormones. In: Kazda, S. & Denenberg, V.H., eds, The Postnatal Development of Phenotype, Prague, Academia, pp. 229-251

US Code of Federal Regulations (1973) Washington DC, US Government Printing Office, 21 CFR 121.245, 121.257, 135 g. 30, 135 g. 38

US Tariff Commission (1973) Imports of Benzenoid Chemicals and Products, 1972, TC Publication 601, Washington DC, US Government Printing Office, p. 85

Woodruff, L.M. (1941) Tumors produced by estradiol benzoate in the guinea pig. Cancer Res., 1, 367-370

OESTRIOL

1. Chemical and Physical Data

1.1 Synonyms and trade names*

Chem. Abstr. No.: 50-27-1

Estra-1,3,5(10)-triene-3,16α,17β-triol; oestra-1,3,5(10)-triene-3, 16α,17β-triol; 1,3,5-estratriene-3β,16α,17β-triol; 1,3,5-oestra-triene-3β,16α,17β-triol; estratriol; oestratriol; estriol; (16α, 17β)-estra-1,3,5(10)-triene-3,16,17-triol; (16α,17β)-oestra-1,3,5(10)-triene-3,16,17-triol; 16α,17β-estriol; 16α,17β-oestriol; 3,16α,17β-estriol; 3,16α,17β-oestriol; follicular hormone hydrate; 16α-hydroxyestradiol; 16α-hydroxyoestradiol; OE_3; 3,16α,17β-trihydroxy-$\Delta^{1,3,5}$-estratriene; 3,16α,17β-trihydroxy-$\Delta^{1,3,5}$-oestratriene; 3,16α, 17β-trihydroxyestra-1,3,5(10)-triene; 3,16α,17β-trihydroxyoestra-1,3, 5(10)-triene; trihydroxyestrin; trihydroxyoestrin

Aacifemine; Colpovister; Destriol; Gynaesan; Hormonin; Ovesterin; Ovestin; Ovestinon; Synapause; Theelol; Tridestrin; Triovex

1.2 Chemical formula and molecular weight

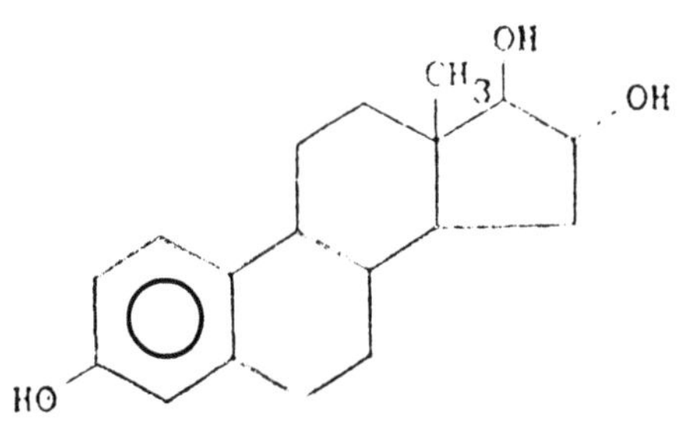

$C_{18}H_{24}O_3$

Mol. wt: 288.4

---

* Trade names include mixtures containing oestriol

1.3 Chemical and physical properties of the pure substance

(a) *Description*: White, very small, monoclinic crystals (from dilute alcohol)

(b) *Melting-point*: 282°C

(c) *Absorption spectrometry*: λ_{max} 280 nm

(d) *Optical rotation*: $\{\alpha\}_D^{25}$ +58° ± 5° (4% w/v in dioxane)

(e) *Solubility*: Practically insoluble in water; soluble at 25°C in 95% ethanol (1 part in 500); soluble in chloroform, dioxane, ether, pyridine, vegetable oils and aqueous solutions of alkali hydroxides

1.4 Technical products and impurities

Oestriol is available in the United States in the form of capsules and as tablets in combinations with oestradiol-17β and oestrone (Kastrup, 1973).

2. Production, Use, Occurrence and Analysis

2.1 Production and use[1]

Isolation of oestriol from the urine of pregnant women was first reported by Marrian (1929). An extraction and crystallization process patented in 1934 (US 1,967,350-1, assigned to St. Louis University) was used commercially for the isolation of oestriol from pregnant mares' urine for several years; however, the present US manufacturer of oestriol is believed to produce it by chemical synthesis. In one, older method, oestrone methyl ether is converted to its 16-oximino derivative, which on reduction and hydrolysis gives the 16-keto-17-hydroxy compound. Reduction of this with sodium and alcohol followed by treatment with hydrobromic acid in acetic acid gives oestriol in low yields. In a more recent, improved method, oestrone acetate is converted to its enol acetate with isopropenyl acetate, and treatment of the enol acetate with perbenzoic acid followed by reduction

---

[1] Data from Chemical Information Services, Stanford Research Institute, USA

with lithium aluminium hydride produces oestriol. No information is available on the method used by the US producing company or on the quantity of oestriol produced.

Oestriol is used alone and in combinations with oestrone and oestradiol for the treatment of kraurosis, menopausal syndrome, pruritis and senile vaginitis (Kastrup, 1973). Total US sales of oestriol for use in human medicine are estimated to be less than 10 kg annually. Oestriol is not known to be used in veterinary medicine.

Data on production of oestriol in the countries of Western Europe are not available, but it is believed that one company in The Netherlands manufactures the chemical. Total sales of oestriol in hormone specialties in Western Europe in 1972 are estimated to have been less than 15 kg. Sales in The Netherlands represented approximately 30% of the total, with lesser amounts sold in Belgium, the Federal Republic of Germany, France, Italy, Spain and the United Kingdom.

2.2 Occurrence

Oestriol is a widely-occurring natural oestrogen (see section, "General Remarks on Sex Hormones", p. 30, for further information). It is also reported to occur in pussywillows (flowers of Salix viminalis) (Merck & Co., 1968).

2.3 Analysis

General methods of analysis are summarized in the section, "General Remarks on the Sex Hormones", p. 40.

3. Biological Data Relevant to the Evaluation of Carcinogenic Risk to Man

3.1 Carcinogenicity and related studies in animals

No long-term carcinogenicity tests were available to the Working Group at the time of the meeting.

3.2 Other relevant biological data

See section, "General Remarks on the Sex Hormones", and pp. 38-40.

3.3 Observations in man

See section, "Oestrogens and Progestins in Relation to Human Cancer", p. 219.

4. Comments on Data Reported and Evaluation[1]

4.1 Animal data

Since oestriol has not been adequately tested in experimental animals, no assessment can be made.

4.2 Human data

No case reports or epidemiological studies were available to the Working Group. Epidemiological studies on steroid hormones used in oestrogen treatment have been summarized in the section, "Oestrogens and Progestins in Relation to Human Cancer", p. 219.

---

[1] This section should be read in conjunction with the section "General Conclusions on Hormones", p. 235.

5. References

Kastrup, E.K., ed. (1973) Facts and Comparisons, St. Louis, Missouri, Facts & Comparisons Inc.

Marrian, G.F. (1929) The chemistry of oestrin. I. Preparation from urine and separation from an unidentified solid alcohol. Biochem. J., 23, 1090-1098

Merck & Co. (1968) The Merck Index, 8th ed., Rahway, N.J., p. 424

OESTRONE

1. Chemical and Physical Data

1.1 Synonyms and trade names*

Chem. Abstr. No.: 53-16-7

1,3,5(10)-Estratrien-3-ol-17-one; 1,3,5(10)-oestratrien-3-ol-17-one; estrone; follicular hormone; 3-hydroxy-17-keto-estra-1,3,5-triene; 3-hydroxy-17-keto-oestra-1,3,5-triene; Δ-1,3,5-estratrien-3β-ol-17-one; Δ-1,3,5-oestratrien-3β-ol-17-one; 3-hydroxy-1,3,5(10)-estratrien-17-one; 3-hydroxy-1,3,5(10)-oestratrien-17-one; 3-hydroxy-estra-1,3,5(10)-trien-17-one; 3-hydroxy-oestra-1,3,5(10)-trien-17-one; theelin; thelykinin

Aquarcrine; Crinovaryl; Cristallovar; Crystogen; Destrone; Disynformon; Endofolliculina; Estrol; Estrone-A; Estrugenone; Estrusol; Femestrone-injection; Femidyn; Folikrin; Folipex; Folisan; Follestrine; Folliculin; Follicunodis; Follidrin; Glandubolin; Harmogen; Hiestrone; Hormofollin; Hormonin; Hormovarine; Kestrone; Ketodestrin; Ketohydroxyestrin; Klimakton; Menagen; Menformon; Oestrin; Oestroform; Oestroperos; Ovex (tablets); Ovifollin; Percutacrine Oest.; Percutacrine Lut.; Perlatan; Proluton D; Solliculin; Templodine; Thelestrin; Thynestron; Trioestrine; Unden; Wynestron

1.2 Chemical formula and molecular weight

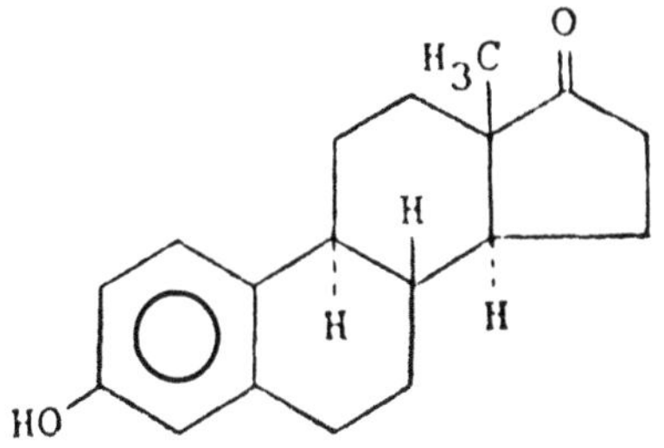

$C_{18}H_{22}O_2$

Mol. wt: 270.4

---

* Trade names include mixtures containing oestrone

1.3 Chemical and physical properties of the pure substance

(a) Description: White crystals (from acetone)
(b) Melting-point: d-form (natural), 254.5-256°C; dl-form (from acetone), 251-254°C
(c) Absorption spectrometry: λ_{max} 283-285 nm
(d) Optical rotation: $\{\alpha\}_D^{25}$ +158° to +168° (1% w/v in dioxane)
$\{\alpha\}_D^{22}$ +152° (0.995% w/v in chloroform)
(e) Solubility: 3 mg in 100 ml water at 25°C; 1 g in 250 ml 96% ethanol at 15°C, in 50 ml boiling ethanol, in 50 ml acetone at 15°C, in 33 ml boiling acetone, in 110 ml chloroform at 15°C, in 80 ml boiling chloroform; soluble in dioxane and aqueous solutions of alkali hydroxides; slightly soluble in ether and vegetable oils.

1.4 Technical products and impurities

Oestrone is available for intramuscular or subcutaneous administration in the form of an aqueous suspension. It is also present as the main component of a mixture of oestrogenic substances which is available as an aqueous suspension and in oil. Three derivatives of oestrone are also produced: (1) sodium oestrone sulphate, which constitutes 50-65% of the water-soluble conjugated oestrogens (20-35% of sodium equilin sulphate is also present) and is sold as such or in combinations with a variety of other drugs (e.g., tranquillizers); (2) piperazine oestrone sulphate, in the form of tablets; and (3) potassium oestrone sulphate, in combinations with oestrone or oestrogenic substances in the form of injections (Kastrup, 1973).

2. Production, Use, Occurrence and Analysis

2.1 Production and use[1]

Isolation of oestrone was first reported by Butenandt (1929) and Doisy

---

[1] Data from Chemical Information Services, Stanford Research Institute, USA

et al. (1929), and the first total synthesis was reported by Anner & Miescher (1948). Several methods of partial synthesis from steroids such as cholesterol and ergosterol were subsequently developed.

In one method, $\Delta^{1,4,6}$-androstatriene-3,17-dione (which is obtained from diosgenin) is pyrolyzed to give 6-dehydro-oestrone, which is catalytically reduced to oestrone. The only US manufacturer of oestrone is believed to produce it by isolation from pregnant mares' urine rather than by chemical synthesis. Pregnant mares' urine is also used by another US company as the source of the so-called "oestrogenic substance" (which contains oestrone as the main component) and of the water-soluble conjugated oestrogens (which contain the oestrone derivative, sodium oestrone sulphate). No data are available on the total US production of oestrone and these related compounds.

Oestrone in its various forms is used in human medicine for the treatment of such conditions as amenorrhea, breast carcinoma, hypogenitalism, menopausal syndrome, postmenopausal osteoporosis, postpartum breast engorgement, prostatic carcinoma and senile vaginitis. In such applications it is frequently used in combinations with other homones, e.g., androgens, other oestrogens and progestins, and sometimes with other medicinals, e.g., barbiturates and tranquillizers (Kastrup, 1973). Total US sales of oestrone in its various forms for use in human medicine are estimated to be less than 2000 kg annually, with the "oestrogenic substance" constituting the largest percentage of the total.

Data on production of oestrone in the countries of Western Europe are not available, but production and sales are known to be concentrated in a small number of companies. Total sales of oestrone in hormone specialties in Western Europe in 1972 are estimated to have been less than 10 kg. Sales in Spain represented approximately 65% of the total, with lesser amounts sold in France and the United Kingdom.

Veterinary uses of oestrone are reported to include replacement therapy in underdeveloped females, treatment of incontinence and vaginitis of spayed bitches, treatment of reproductive disorders and other conditions. It is used to induce oestrus or ovulation (Merck & Co., 1968).

Oestrone may also be used as an intermediate in the synthesis of other oestrogens (e.g., oestradiol-17β and oestriol), but the quantity used for this purpose is not known.

2.2 Occurrence

Oestrone is a widely-occurring natural oestrogen (see section, "General Remarks on the Sex Hormones", p. 30, for further information). It is also reportedly found in palm-kernel oil (Merck & Co., 1968).

2.3 Analysis

General methods of analysis are summarized in the section "General Remarks on Sex Hormones", p. 40.

3. Biological Data Relevant to the Evaluation of Carcinogenic Risk to Man

3.1 Carcinogenicity and related studies in animals

(a) Oral administration

Mouse: Boot & Muhlbock (1956) found that 125 µg/l oestrone in the drinking-water resulted in the appearance of breast tumours in 33/68 gonadectomized male C3H mice freed of the mammary tumour virus (MTV). At a concentration of 2000 µg/l, the incidence of mammary tumours increased to 119/169. {These data are difficult to assess in view of the fact that gonadectomy alone results in adrenal hypertrophy, which gives rise to oestrogenic stimulation without other treatment.}

(b) Subcutaneous and/or intramuscular injection

Mouse: Lacassagne (1932) first reported the induction of mammary tumours in 3/3 male mice of the RIII strain (with the MTV) after weekly injections (not specified) of 0.6 mg oestrone benzoate for more than 5 months. Lacassagne (1939) also demonstrated the role of the maternal influence (i.e., transmission of the milk-borne MTV) by crossing RIII strain mice, which have a high incidence in untreated females, with strain 39 mice, which have no spontaneous mammary tumour incidence. Injection (not specified) of 50 µg oestrone benzoate weekly induced tumours of the breast only in male hybrids whose mothers came from the high mammary tumour incidence strain (RIII). Males with a strain 39 mother and an RIII father had no mammary tumours with this treatment.

Bonser (1936) found breast tumours in 3/21 male A strain mice (with the MTV) but in none of 40 CBA males (lacking the MTV) after weekly s.c. injections of 300-500 units (30-50 µg) oestrone benzoate in oil for 43 weeks or more. Shimkin & Grady (1940) induced breast tumours in 2/10 male C3H mice (with the MTV) by the s.c. injection of 50 µg oestrone in oil weekly for 24 weeks. Similar treatment of female C3H mice reduced the average age at the appearance of mammary cancer from 46 weeks in untreated controls to 30 weeks in the treated animals. In both groups of females the incidence of tumours was 100%.

Rat: Injection of large amounts of oestrone (50-200 µg) daily in oil (total dose, 30-40 mg) induced breast cancers in 6/6 castrated male rats and in 4/5 ovariectomized females (Geschickter & Byrnes, 1942). A lower incidence was found in intact males (2/6) and in intact females (3/8). The average induction time ranged from 83 weeks at the lowest dosage to 31 weeks at the highest dosage. Chamorro (1943) induced mammary cancer in 1/2 male and 5/8 female rats given twice weekly s.c. injections of 50-100 µg oestrone benzoate in oil for 20 months. Pituitary tumours (140-271 mg in weight) were present in all rats.

Hamster: Dontenwill (1958) found malignant kidney tumours of different structures in 43/86 unilaterally nephrectomized, castrated male golden hamsters injected with oestrone (dose not stated) after 8 months. Pituitary adenomas also occurred in about 25% of the animals.

(c) Subcutaneous implantation (pellets)

Mouse: Bittner (1941) implanted 2 mg pellets of oestrone s.c. in mice of the A and C3H strains when the animals were 4-6 weeks of age. Breast tumours arose both in treated A males and in C3H and A females carrying the MTV, but not in mice fostered by C57BL females nor in strains from which the MTV was excluded. He concluded that oestrone treatment was not as effective in tumour induction in females as was forced breeding.

Mice of various hybrids between the A, C3H, C57 and JK strains which were implanted with pellets of oestrone (1-7 mg) had an overall incidence of lymphoid tumours of 19/105 compared to 21/391 in corresponding control mice (Gardner & Dougherty, 1944).

Rat: Dunning et al. (1953) reported tumours of the breast in A x C rats (3/32 females, 4/30 males), Fischer rats (3/29 females, 2/29 males) and August rats (5/12 females, 9/25 males) implanted with a single pellet of oestrone (8-12 mg); average latency periods ranged from 51-97 weeks. Breast cancer incidence was doubled in A x C rats by the implantation of two such pellets, and the latent period was reduced by 50%. Adrenal cortical tumours were found in small numbers of rats with one pellet, but the incidence was greatly reduced with two pellets. No breast tumours were seen in either sex of rats of the Copenhagen strain, but 6 males and 1 female had bladder cancer associated with bladder stones. The amount of oestrone absorbed was calculated to be between 3.5 and 9.4 mg per rat. There was no control group. {The occurrence of the bladder stones is attributable to the oestrone treatment, but the occurrence of bladder cancer is probably attributable to the presence of stones and not directly to the oestrone.}

Noble (1967) found adrenal cortical tumours in 20% of female hooded rats implanted with pellets of oestrone (dose not stated). The tumours frequently metastasized and were transplantable, but they regressed if the oestrone treatment was withdrawn. Adrenal tumours occurred in about 5% of untreated rats in that colony.

Cutts (1966) summarized extensive experiments on mammary tumour induction by s.c. implanted pellets of oestrone (average, 10 mg). The incidences of breast tumours in females of different strains after 43-57 weeks of treatment were: Fischer, 16%; Wistar, 24%; Lewis, 38%; Sprague-Dawley, 42%; and hooded, 86%. The estimated absorption of oestrone was between 6 and 7 µg/day. There was no control group.

Hamster: Kirkman (1959) reported that the implantation of 20 mg pellets of oestrone induced malignant kidney tumours (not specified) in 7/8 intact male Syrian hamsters and in 10/10 castrates. There were no kidney tumours in 61 intact or in 60 castrated males.

(d) Skin application

Mouse: Cramer & Horning (1936) reported the induction of breast tumours in 5/5 male mice of the RIII strain (carrying the MTV) after skin application of oestrone as a 0.01% solution in chloroform twice weekly for 16 or more weeks. Female RIII mice had no breast tumours following the same treatment for more than 6 months, although the incidence in untreated females was 60-70%. Three pituitary tumours were observed among 12 mice of both sexes treated with oestrone. In a mixed strain of mice with a low incidence of breast tumours, no mammary cancers were induced by oestrone treatment after 44 weeks.

(e) Other experimental systems

Intravaginal implantation: Oestrone pellets weighing 40 mg were fixed intravaginally in 30 golden hamsters. Carcinoma of the vagina and cervix developed in 6/9 animals alive after 14 months (Dontenwill et al., 1963). {The method was complicated by mechanical difficulties and by inflammatory reactions.}

3.2 Other relevant biological data

See section, "General Remarks on the Sex Hormones", and pp. 38-40.

3.3 Observations in man

See section, "Oestrogens and Progestins in Relation to Human Cancer", p. 219.

4. Comments on Data Reported and Evaluation[1]

4.1 Animal data

Oestrone was tested orally in mice; by subcutaneous injection and by implantation in mice, rats and hamsters; and by skin-painting in mice. Its administration resulted in an increased incidence of mammary tumours in mice;

---

[1] This section should be read in conjunction with the section, "General Conclusions on Hormones", p. 235.

in pituitary, adrenal and mammary tumours and bladder tumours in association with stones in rats; and in renal tumours in both castrated and intact male hamsters.

Oestrone treatment increased the incidence of mammary tumours in strains of mice having a spontaneous incidence of the tumours which may be related to the presence of a virus. No evidence of a possible role of a virus has been demonstrated in rats.

4.2 Human data

No case reports or epidemiological studies were available to the Working Group. Epidemiological studies on steroid hormones used in oestrogen treatment have been summarized in the section, "Oestrogens and Progestins in Relation to Human Cancer", p. 219.

5. References

Anner, G. & Miescher, K. (1948) Die Synthese des natürlichen Oestrons. Totalsynthesen in der Oestronreihe. III. Helv. chim. Acta., 31, 2173-2183

Bittner, J.J. (1941) The influence of estrogens on the incidence of tumors in foster nursed mice. Cancer Res., 1, 290-292

Bonser, G.M. (1936) The effect of oestrone administration on the mammary glands of male mice of two strains differing greatly in their susceptibility to spontaneous mammary carcinoma. J. Path. Bact., 42, 169-181

Boot, L.M. & Mühlbock, O. (1956) The mammary tumour incidence in the C3H mouse strain with and without the agent (C3H, $C3H_f$, $C3H_e$). Acta Un. int. Cancr., 12, 569-581

Butenandt, A. (1929) Über "Progynon" ein krystallisiertes weibliches Sexualhormon. Naturwissenschaften, 17, 879

Chamorro, A. (1943) Production par le benzoate d'oestrone d'adénocarcinome mammaire chez des rats. C.R. Soc. Biol. (Paris), 137, 325-326

Cramer, W. & Horning, E.S. (1936) Experimental production by oestrin of pituitary tumours with hypopituitarism and of mammary cancer. Lancet, i, 247-249

Cutts, J.H. (1966) Estrogen-induced breast cancer in the rat. Canad. Cancer Conf., 6, 50-68

Doisy, E.A., Veler, C.D. & Thayer, S. (1929) Folliculin from urine of pregnant women. Amer. J. Physiol., 90, 329-330

Dontenwill, W. (1958) Experimentelle Erzeugung von Nieren- und Lebertumoren durch Follikelhormon. Verh. Dtsch. Ges. Path., 42, 458-461

Dontenwill, W., Mohr, U. & Bernhard, J. (1963) Die unterschiedliche Wirkung des Follikelhormons auf die Portio- und Vaginalschleimhaut bei parenteraler und lokaler Applikation. Z. Krebsforsch., 65, 303-308

Dunning, W.F., Curtis, M.R. & Segaloff, A. (1953) Strain differences in response to estrone and the induction of mammary gland, adrenal and bladder cancer in rats. Cancer Res., 13, 147-152

Gardner, W.U. & Dougherty, T.F. (1944) The leukemogenic action of estrogens in hybrid mice. Yale J. Biol. Med., 17, 75-90

Geschickter, C.F. & Byrnes, E.W. (1942) Factors influencing the development and time of appearance of mammary cancer in the rat in response to estrogen. Arch. Path., 33, 334-356

Kastrup, E.K., ed. (1973) Facts and Comparisons, St. Louis, Missouri, Facts & Comparisons Inc.

Kirkman, H. (1959) Estrogen-induced tumors of the kidney. IV. Incidence in female Syrian hamsters. Nat. Cancer Inst. Monogr., 1, 59-75

Lacassagne, A. (1932) Apparition de cancers de la mamelle chez la souris mâle, soumise à des injections de folliculine. C.R. Acad. Sci. (Paris), 195, 630-632

Lacassagne, A. (1939) Confirmation, par des expériences de traitement à l'oestrone, du rôle prépondérant de la mère dans la transmission héréditaire du carcinome de la mamelle. C.R. Soc. Biol. (Paris), 132, 222-224

Merck & Co. (1968) The Merck Index, 8th ed., Rahway, N.J., p. 424

Noble, R.L. (1967) Induced transplantable estrogen-dependent carcinoma of the adrenal cortex in rats. Proc. Amer. Ass. Cancer Res., 8, 51

Shimkin, M.B. & Grady, H.G. (1940) Carcinogenic potency of stilbestrol and estrone in strain C3H mice. J. nat. Cancer Inst., 1, 119-128

PROGESTINS

PROGESTERONE

1. Chemical and Physical Data

1.1 Synonyms and trade names*

Chem. Abstr. No.: 57-83-0

Corpus luteum hormone; luteal hormone; luteohormone; luteine; pregn-4-en-3,20-dione; 3,20-pregnene-4; pregnenedione; pregnene-3,20-dione; pregn-4-ene-3,20-dione; Δ^4-pregnene-3,20-dione; 4-pregnene-3,20-dione; β-progesterone; progesteronum; progestin

Corlutin; Corlutina; Corluvite; Corporin; Cycloestrol; Duogynon; Emmenovis; Emonovister; Farlutal; Flavolutan; Foliluteina; Fologenon; Gestone; Gestormone; Glanducorpin; Hormoflaveine; Hormoluton; Lipo-lutin; Lucorteum sol; Luteinique; Luteocrin; Luteodyn; Luteo Folicular; Luteogan; Luteogyl; Luteol; Luteosan; Luteostab; Luteovis; Lutestex; Lutestron; Lutex; Lutidon; Lutocycli Lutocyclin M; Lutocylin; Lutoform; Lutogyl; Lutovitamina E; Lut Ovociclina; Lut-ovocyclin; Lutren; Lutrogen; Lutromone; Lutrone; Nalutron; Percutacrine Lut.; Piaponon; Precyclan-Leo; Primolut; Progekan; Progesterol; Progesterone R; Progestilline Fort; Progestogel; Progestone; Prolidon; Proluton; Proluton D; Proluton Dep.; Proluton-Oestradiol; Proluton Z; Protectona; Stroluten; Synergon; Syngesterone; Synovex S; Syntoluton; Testo Luteinica; Testoluton; Testoviron Prog.; Tocogestan; Trioestrine; Trioestrine R; Trioestrine Vitam.; Vit-E-Progesterone

---

* Trade names include mixtures containing progesterone

1.2 Chemical formula and molecular weight

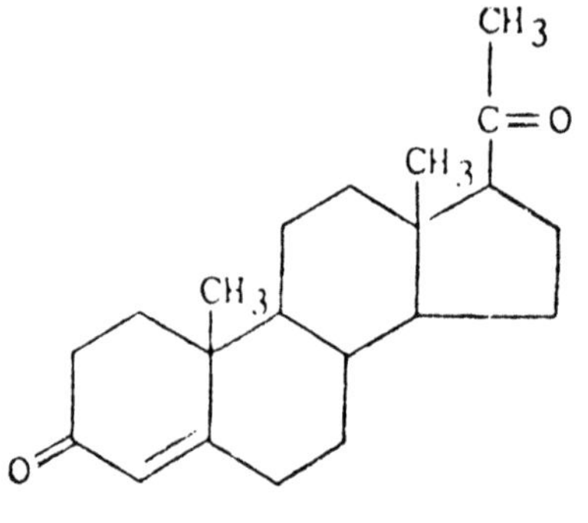

$C_{21}H_{30}O_2$

Mol. wt: 314.5

1.3 Chemical and physical properties of the pure substance

(a) Description: Exists in two readily interconvertible forms:-

α-form - white orthorhombic crystals
β-form - white orthorhombic needles

(b) Melting-point: α-form - 127-131°C
β-form - 121°C

(c) Absorption spectrometry: λ_{max} 240 nm

(d) Optical rotation: $\{\alpha\}_D^{20}$ +172° to +182° (2% w/v in dioxane)

(e) Solubility: Practically insoluble in water; soluble at 25°C in 95% ethanol (1 in 8), arachis oil (1 in 60), chloroform (1 in 0.33), ether (1 in 16), ethyl acetate (1 in 60), light petroleum (1 in 100); also soluble in acetone, benzene, dioxane and oils

1.4 Technical products and impurities

Progesterone is available in the United States in the form of injections, as an aqueous suspension and as a solution in vegetable oil. Combinations of progesterone and oestrogenic substance are also available, in the form of tablets and of injections of aqueous suspensions and oil solutions (Kastrup, 1973).

2. Production, Use, Occurrence and Analysis

2.1 Production and use[1]

Isolation of progesterone was first reported by Butenandt & Westphal (1934) and by Wintersteiner & Allen (1934); numerous methods of synthesis from other steroids (e.g., cholesterol and stigmasterol) were subsequently reported. One of the two US manufacturers of progesterone is believed to produce it from intermediates obtained by the degradation of diosgenin. In one method, degradation produces pregnenolone, which is converted to progesterone by Oppenauer oxidation. The other US manufacturer of progesterone is believed to produce it from intermediates derived from stigmasterol.

Until about 1944 world production of progesterone was only a few kg per year, and even in 1951 it was less than 1 000 kg. However, in 1952 one Mexican manufacturer alone produced over 9 000 kg (Anon., 1967). The present annual production of the two US manufacturers is not known.

In the past progesterone was recommended for use in the treatment of a large number of menstrual disorders, e.g., abnormal uterine bleeding due to hormonal imbalance, ammenorrhea, habitual abortion and threatened abortion. However, in some of these applications it has been displaced by orally active progestins, and its efficacy in other uses has been put into question. In October 1973 the US Food and Drug Administration proposed to restrict the approved uses of progesterone injection to the treatment of amenorrhea and of abnormal uterine bleeding due to hormonal imbalance, in the absence of organic pathology such as submucous fibroids or uterine cancer (US Environmental Protection Agency, 1973). Combinations of progesterone with oestrogenic substances (as injections or tablets) are used for the treatment of secondary amenorrhea or of functional uterine bleeding (Kastrup, 1973). Prior to the recent governmental action, total US sales of progesterone for use in human medicine were estimated to have been less than 50 kg annually.

---

[1] Data from Chemical Information Services, Stanford Research Institute, USA

Data on production of progesterone in the countries of Western Europe are not available, but it is believed that one company in France manufactures the chemical. Total sales of progesterone in hormone specialties in Western Europe in 1972 are estimated to have been less than 500 kg. Sales in France represented approximately 60% of the total, with lesser amounts sold in Belgium, the Federal Republic of Germany, Italy, The Netherlands and Spain.

Subcutaneous ear implants of combinations of progesterone and oestradiol benzoate are approved in the US for the promotion of growth and feed efficiency in lambs and steers (US Code of Federal Regulations, 1973), and the quantity of progesterone used for this purpose may have increased in recent months as a result of the US Food and Drug Administration ban on the use of diethylstilboestrol implants as a growth promoter for these animals.

Veterinary uses of progesterone include control of habitual abortion in cattle and delay of oestrus and ovulation in cattle, pigs and dogs (Merck & Co., 1968). No data are available on the quantity of progesterone consumed in the US for veterinary purposes.

2.2 Occurrence

Progesterone is a widely-occurring, natural progestin (see section, "General Remarks on the Sex Hormones", p. 30, for further information).

2.3 Analysis

General methods of analysis are summarized in the section, "General Remarks on the Sex Hormones", p. 40.

3. Biological Data Relevant to the Evaluation of Carcinogenic Risk of Man

3.1 Carcinogenicity and related studies in animals

(a) Subcutaneous and/or intramuscular injection

Mouse: Burrows & Hoch-Ligeti (1946) found that up to 34 weekly s.c. injections of 1 mg progesterone in arachis oil did not increase the incidence of breast tumours in 30 female C3H mice compared with that in 20 controls; however, the incidence was very high in both the treated and control groups, and tumours occurred at an early age. {This may have obscured any effect, and the age at the start of treatment was also quite advanced. Similar reservations apply to the results of Heiman (1945), who used RIII mice.}

Jull (1954) found that s.c. administration of 0.5 µg progesterone every two weeks combined with 50 µg oestradiol dipropionate in oil given once a week to ovariectomized IF mice increased the incidence of tumours induced by 3-methylcholanthrene compared to that produced by oestrogen only plus the carcinogen (the respective incidences were 9/11 and 2/20). Similar but less significant results were found in male mice, the incidences being 4/14 and 1/29.

Kaslaris & Jull (1962) found that 10 mg progesterone injected s.c. in arachis oil weekly until death reduced the induction of adenocarcinomas in the uterine horns of mature ovariectomized CBA mice exposed to local implants of 0.1 mg 3-methylcholanthrene from 23 to 0%; however, there was a corresponding increase from 3 to 31% in the incidence of connective tissue tumours.

Poel (1965) found that 2.5 mg progesterone in peanut oil given s.c. 5 times weekly for 19 weeks increased the incidence of breast tumours induced by 3-methylcholanthrene (MCA) in C3H female mice (with the MTV) to 23/23, compared with 5/24 for MCA alone and 2/25 for progesterone alone. A similar action of progesterone with MCA was observed in groups of 26-28 C3H mice without the MTV, although the effect in this case was mainly to shorten the latent period from 40 to 25 weeks. When progesterone alone was administered to C3H mice with the MTV the incidence of breast tumours was increased from 6/24 with vehicle only to 21/24, and the latent period was diminished from 70 to 55 weeks. Progesterone alone given to 27 C3H mice without the MTV did not induce tumours within 42 weeks (Poel, 1968; 1969).

Glucksmann & Cherry (1962) reported that the incidence of mixed carcinomas of the cervix or vagina in female C3H mice given weekly intravaginal applications of a 1% solution of 9,10-dimethyl-1,2-benzanthracene (DMBA) was increased by ovariectomy. The incidence of mixed carcinomas in ovariectomized,

DMBA-treated mice was 3/8 (38%), compared with 0/17 in intact, DMBA-treated mice; and squamous-cell carcinomas of the cervix or vagina occurred in 5/15 ovariectomized mice, compared with 13/17 (76%) intact mice. In a group of 16 ovariectomized C3H females given the DMBA treatment together with twice-weekly i.m. injections of 0.2 mg progesterone, the incidence of squamous-cell carcinomas reached 13/16 (81%), and mixed carcinomas occurred in 5/16 (31%) mice.

Rat: In rats, progesterone injected s.c. or i.m. at doses of 3-4 mg/day decreased the latent period and/or increased the incidence of breast tumours induced by single doses of 20 mg DMBA or of 10 mg MCA, but only when injections were commenced after administration of the carcinogen (Huggins et al., 1959; Huggins & Yang, 1962; Jabara et al., 1973). In other experiments, where progesterone was injected for varying periods before administration of a carcinogen, the resulting incidence of breast tumours was significantly diminished from 13/20 to 6/16 (Jull, 1966; Briziarelli, 1966; Welsch et al., 1968; Jabara et al., 1973). Other experiments, in which progesterone was injected s.c. together with an oestrogen after dosage with DMBA, are difficult to interpret due to the known inhibitory effects of oestrogens on mammary carcinogenesis (McCormick & Moon, 1973). It has been shown that oestrogen treatment of ovariectomized female rats is not sufficient to restore susceptibility to mammary carcinogenesis by MCA; however, treatment with a combination of progesterone with oestrogen i.m. is a sufficient replacement for the ovaries (Sydnor & Cockrell, 1963). Cantarow et al. (1948) reported an increase from 17/57 to 22/26 in the incidence of breast tumours in female rats fed 0.03% 2-acetylaminofluorene in the diet and injected i.m. with 0.5 mg progesterone 3 times weekly for life.

Progesterone (0.3 mg) injected s.c. 3 times weekly for 21 weeks increased the latent period of induction of breast tumours in female hooded rats by oestrone from 37 to 50 weeks but did not change the incidence of mammary tumours (Cutts, 1964).

In intact rats, i.m. injections of progesterone (1 mg twice weekly) retarded by approximately 4 weeks the induction of sarcomas of the cervix and vagina produced by local application of 1% DMBA in acetone weekly for life, but the induction of papillomas was promoted by 19 weeks. Progesterone alone did not increase the rate of carcinogenesis in ovariectomized rats treated with the carcinogen; however, when it was combined with oestrogen, the incidence but not the latent period of tumour induction was restored to that of intact females (Glucksman & Cherry, 1968).

Rabbit: 10 mg progesterone injected s.c. twice weekly into 32 rabbits exposed to vaginal strings containing 3-methylcholanthrene did not affect the incidence of vaginal tumours occurring within 20 months, the incidences being 5/23 in controls compared with 4/31 in treated animals (Alvizouri & Ramiréz de Pita, 1964).

Dog: Long-term s.c. injections of progesterone for a total of 74 weeks, increasing in dosage from 0.08 to 22.5 mg daily, caused endometrial hyperplasia, inhibition of ovarian development and marked mammary hyperplasia in female beagle dogs. No tumours were reported in animals killed 24 hours after the last dose, but fibro-adenomatous nodules occurred in 2/5 dogs given the highest doses of progesterone (Capel-Edwards et al., 1973).

(b) Subcutaneous implantation

Mouse: Trentin (1954) implanted high doses of progesterone (14 mg pellets every 28 days during 104 weeks) s.c. in 59 female C3H x A hybrid mice (with the MTV) and found breast carcinomas at a significantly earlier age and in a higher incidence (88% at 70 weeks) than among 58 untreated control mice (62% at 93 weeks). No mammary tumours appeared among 27 intact or among 24 castrated, untreated, male controls or in 27 progesterone-treated, intact males. However, 2/26 castrated males given progesterone developed mammary tumours.

Lipschütz et al. (1967a) found that the absorption of 29 µg/day or more of progesterone from pellets implanted s.c. was required to suppress corpus luteum formation in the ovaries of mice. After 18 months' treatment with 59-900 µg/day progesterone, so-called ovarian granulosa-cell tumours were found in 27/83 BALB/c mice. Only 3 of these tumours exceeded 5 mm in size, most of them measuring less than 0.5 mm in diameter. One microscopic tumour occurred among 33 control mice killed after 18 months.

Following the absorption from s.c. pellets of 18-900 µg/day progesterone alone, uterine sarcomas were observed in 15/142 mice after a period of 18 months. Most of these tumours were very small, and no tumours were found in 33 controls (Lipschütz et al., 1967b).

A group of 20 female BALB/c mice treated with 5 mg s.c. pellets of a progesterone-cholesterol mixture for an average period of 17 months developed no precancerous or cancerous lesions of the cervix and/or vagina. However, when 39 mice were treated with intravaginal inoculations of herpesvirus type 2 in addition to the progesterone pellets, 1 precancerous lesion and 1 squamous-cell carcinoma of the cervix were observed. No tumours of the cervix or vagina were found in 15 control mice (Muñoz, 1973).

After local applications of the carcinogen 3-methylcholanthrene (MCA) in 50 C57BL6 mice, Reboud & Pageaut (1973) found that 15 mg progesterone implanted s.c. every 3 weeks for 9 weeks increased the incidence of vaginal-cervical invasive squamous-cell carcinomas from 6/50 with MCA alone to 45/50.

Rat: In A x C rats implanted s.c. with 25 mg pellets containing 20 mg progesterone/100 g bw and observed for 40 weeks, an increased incidence of liver-cell carcinomas induced by N-2-fluorenyldiacetamide was observed in intact male rats (11/11 versus 7/12), in castrated males (5/13 versus 1/9) and in ovariectomized females (4/12 versus 0/14), but the treatment did not increase the incidence of these tumours in intact females (0/9 versus 1/10) (Reuber & Firminger, 1962).

In female A x C rats treated with diethylstilboestrol (DES) and/or progesterone (20 mg implanted intrascapularly) plus irradiation, the development of mammary tumours was inhibited in the presence of progesterone. The incidence was reduced from 12/21 with DES + irradiation to 1/21 with DES + progesterone + irradiation; the incidence was 0/11 with progesterone + irradiation (Segaloff, 1973).

3.2 Other relevant biological data

See section, "General Remarks on the Sex Hormones", and pp. 38-40.

3.3 Observations in man

See section, "Oestrogens and Progestins in Relation to Human Cancer", p. 219.

4. Comments on Data Reported and Evaluation[1]

4.1 Animal data

Progesterone was tested by subcutaneous or intramuscular injection in mice, rats, rabbits and dogs and by subcutaneous implantation in mice and rats. It was tested alone only in mice and dogs; in rats and rabbits it was always given in combination with other chemicals; in mice it was also tested in combination with other carcinogens.

When given alone, it increased the incidence of ovarian, uterine or mammary tumours in mice, while the experiment in dogs was of insufficient duration to allow an assessment to be made.

The administration of progesterone to intact or castrated mice and rats and to rabbits in combination with polycyclic aromatic hydrocarbons or with 2-acetylaminofluorene and/or oestrogen variously affected the incidence and the histological type of the tumours produced by these known carcinogens (mainly mammary, uterine and vaginal tumours). In particular, progesterone enhanced the incidence of tumours produced by these known carcinogens, but only when given after and not before their administration.

4.2 Human data

No case reports or epidemiological studies on progesterone were available to the Working Group.

---

[1] This section should be read in conjunction with the section "General Conclusions on Hormones", p. 235.

5. References

Alvizouri, M. & Ramiréz de Pita, V. (1964) Experimental carcinoma of the cervix. Hormonal influences. *Amer. J. Obstet. Gynec.*, 89, 940-945

Anon. (1967) *A corporation and a molecule*, Mexico City, Syntex Corp.

Briziarelli, G. (1966) Effects of hormonal pre-treatment against the induction of mammary tumors by 7,12-dimethylbenz(a)anthracene in rats. *Z. Krebsforsch.*, 68, 217-223

Butenandt, A. & Westphal, U. (1934) Zur Isolierung und Charakterisierung des Corpus-luteum-Hormons. *Ber. dtsch. chem. Ges.*, 67, 1440-1442

Burrows, H. & Hoch-Ligeti, C. (1946) Effects of progesterone on the development of mammary cancer in C3H mice. *Cancer Res.*, 6, 608-609

Cantarow, A., Stasney, J. & Paschkis, K.E. (1948) The influence of sex hormones on mammary tumors induced by 2-acetaminofluorene. *Cancer Res.*, 8, 412-417

Capel-Edwards, K., Hall, D.E., Fellowes, K.P., Vallance, D.K., Davies, M.J., Lamb, D. & Robertson, W.B. (1973) Long-term administration of progesterone to the female beagle dog. *Toxicol appl. Pharmacol.*, 24, 474-488

Cutts, J.H. (1964) Estrone-induced mammary tumors in the rat. II. Effect of alterations in the hormonal environment on tumor induction, behaviour and growth. *Cancer Res.*, 24, 1124-1130

Glucksman, A. & Cherry, C.P. (1962) The effect of castration and of additional hormonal treatments on the induction of cervical and vulval tumours in mice. *Brit. J. Cancer*, 16, 634-652

Glucksman, A. & Cherry, C.P. (1968) The effect of oestrogens, testosterone and progesterone on the induction of cervico-vaginal tumours in intact and castrate rats. *Brit. J. Cancer*, 22, 545-562

Heiman, J. (1945) The effect of progesterone and testosterone propionate on the incidence of mammary cancer in mice. *Cancer Res.*, 5, 426-430

Huggins, C. & Yang, N.C. (1962) Induction and extinction of mammary cancer. *Science*, 137, 257-262

Huggins, C., Briziarelli, G. & Sutton, H., Jr (1959) Rapid induction of mammary carcinoma in the rat and the influence of hormones on the tumors. *J. exp. Med.*, 109, 25-42

Jabara, A.G., Toyne, P.H. & Harcourt, A.G. (1973) Effects of time and duration of progesterone administration on mammary tumours induced by 7,12-dimethylbenz(a)anthracene in Sprague-Dawley rats. Brit. J. Cancer, 27, 63-71

Jull, J.W. (1954) The effects of oestrogens and progesterone on the chemical induction of mammary cancer in mice of the IF strain. J. Path. Bact., 68, 547-559

Jull, J.W. (1966) The effect of infection, hormonal environment and genetic constitution on mammary tumor induction in rats by 7,12-dimethylbenz(a)anthracene. Cancer Res., 26, 2368-2373

Kaslaris, E. & Jull, J.W. (1962) The induction of tumours following the direct implantation of four chemical carcinogens into the uterus of mice and the effect of strain and hormones thereon. Brit. J. Cancer, 16, 479-483

Kastrup, E.K., ed. (1973) Facts and Comparisons, St. Louis, Missouri, Facts & Comparisons Inc.

Lipschütz, A., Iglesias, R., Panasevich, V.I. & Salinas, S. (1967a) Granulosa-cell tumours induced in mice by progesterone. Brit. J. Cancer, 21, 144-152

Lipschütz, A., Iglesias, R., Panasevich, V.I. & Salinas, S. (1967b) Pathological changes induced in the uterus of mice with the prolonged administration of progesterone and 19-nor-contraceptives. Brit. J. Cancer, 21, 160-165

McCormick, G.M. & Moon, R.C. (1973) Effect of increasing doses of estrogen and progesterone on mammary carcinogenesis in the rat. Europ. J. Cancer, 9, 483-486

Merck & Co. (1968) The Merck Index, 8th ed., Rahway, N.J., p. 868

Muñoz, N. (1973) Effect of herpesvirus type 2 and hormonal imbalance on the uterine cervix of the mouse. Cancer Res., 33, 1504-1508

Poel, W.E. (1965) Progesterone and the prolonged progestational state: co-carcinogenic factors in mammary tumor induction. Brit. J. Cancer, 19, 824-829

Poel, W.E. (1968) Progesterone enhancement of mammary tumor development as a model of co-carcinogenesis. Brit. J. Cancer, 22, 867-873

Poel, W.E. (1969) Bioassays with inbred mice: their relevance for the random-bred animal. Progr. exp. Tumor Res., 11, 444-460

Reboud, S. & Pageaut, G. (1973) Co-carcinogenic effect of progesterone on 20-methylcholanthrene-induced cervical carcinoma in mice. Nature (Lond.), 241, 398-399

Reuber, M.D. & Firminger, H.I. (1962) Effect of progesterone and diethylstilbestrol on hepatic carcinogenesis and cirrhosis in A x C rats fed N-2-fluorenyldiacetamide. J. nat. Cancer Inst., 29, 933-943

Segaloff, A. (1973) Inhibition by progesterone of radiation-estrogen-induced mammary cancer in the rat. Cancer Res., 33, 1136-1137

Sydnor, K.L. & Cockrell, B. (1963) Influence of estradiol-17β, progesterone and hydrocortisone on 3-methylcholanthrene-induced mammary cancer in intact and ovariectomized Sprague-Dawley rats. Endocrinology, 73, 427-432

Trentin, J.J. (1954) Effect of long-term treatment with high levels of progesterone on the incidence of mammary tumors in mice. Proc. Amer. Ass. Cancer Res., 1, 50

US Code of Federal Regulations (1973) Washington DC, US Government Printing Office, 21 CFR 135 b.4

US Environmental Protection Agency (1973) Medroxyprogesterone acetate; norethindrone; norethindrone acetate; progesterone; diprogesterone; and hydroxyprogesterone caproate. US Federal Register, 38, No. 195, Washington DC, US Government Printing Office, pp. 27947-27949

Welsch, C.W., Clemens, J.A. & Meites, J. (1968) Effects of multiple pituitary homografts or progesterone on 7,12-dimethylbenz(a)anthracene-induced mammary tumors in rats. J. nat. Cancer Inst., 41, 465-471

Wintersteiner, O. & Allen, W.M. (1934) Crystalline progestin. J. biol. Chem., 107, 321-336

17-HYDROXYPROGESTERONES

CHLORMADINONE ACETATE

1. Chemical and Physical Data

1.1 Synonyms and trade names*

Chem. Abstr. No.: 30-22-27

17-Acetoxy-6-chloro-6-dehydroprogesterone; 17α-acetoxy-6-chloro-6-dehydroprogesterone; 17α-acetoxy-6-chloropregna-4,6-diene-3,20-dione; 17-(acetyloxy)-6-chloropregna-4,6-diene-3,20-dione; CAP; chlormadinone; 6-chloro-17-acetoxypregna-4,6-diene-3,20-dione; 6-chloro-17-acetoxy-4,6-pregnadiene-3,20-dione; 6-chloro-17α-acetoxy-4,6-pregnadiene-3,20-dione; Δ^6-6-chloro-17α-acetoxyprogesterone; 6-chloro-Δ^6-17-acetoxyprogesterone; 6-chloro-Δ^6-dehydro-17-acetoxyprogesterone; 6-chloro-6-dehydro-17-acetoxyprogesterone; 6-chloro-6-dehydro-17α-acetoxyprogesterone; 6-chloro-6,7-dehydro-17-acetoxyprogesterone; 6-chloro-6-dehydro-17α-hydroxyprogesterone acetate; 6-chloro-17α-hydroxypregna-4,6-diene-3,20-dione acetate; 6-chloro-17-hydroxy-4,6-pregnadiene-3,20-dione acetate; 6-chloro-17-hydroxypregna-4,6-diene-3,20-dione acetate; 6-chloro-17α-hydroxy-Δ^6-progesterone acetate; 6-chloro-$\Delta^{4,6}$-pregnadien-17α-ol-3,20-dione 17-acetate; 6-chloro-pregna-4,6-dien-17α-ol-3,20-dione acetate; 6-dehydro-6-chloro-17α-acetoxyprogesterone

Aconcen; Anconcene; AY 13390-6; Consan; C-Quens; C-Quens 21; Estirona; Estirona 21; Eunomin; Gestafortin; Gestakliman; Lormin; Luteral; Luteran; Lutestral; Lutoral; Lutinyl; Matrol; Nocon; RS 1280; Sequens; Skedule TM; St 155; Volenyl

---

* Trade names include mixtures containing chlormadinone acetate

1.2 **Chemical formula and molecular weight**

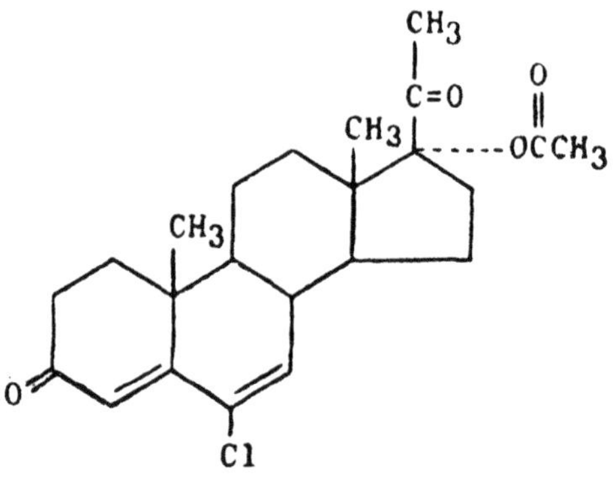

$C_{23}H_{29}ClO_4$

Mol. wt: 404.9

1.3 **Chemical and physical properties of the pure substance**

(a) *Description*: White to creamy-white crystals (from methanol or ether)

(b) *Melting-point*: 212-214°C

(c) *Absorption spectrometry*: λ_{max}283.5 nm (ε = 23,400)
λ_{max}286 nm (ε = 22,100)

(d) *Optical rotation*: $\{\alpha\}_D^{25}$ +6° (1% w/v in chloroform)

(e) *Solubility*: Practically insoluble in water; soluble at 25°C in 95% ethanol (1 in 160), chloroform (1 in 1.5), ether (1 in 210) and methyl alcohol (1 in 130)

1.4 **Technical products and impurities**

Chlormadinone acetate has not been available as a pharmaceutical ingredient in the United States since late 1970, when the only product containing it (an oral contraceptive) was removed from the market after studies by the US Food and Drug Administration showed that breast nodules developed in beagles given high doses of the chemical.

2. Production, Use, Occurrence and Analysis

2.1 Production and use[1]

A method for the synthesis of chlormadinone acetate was first patented in West Germany in 1960 (Ger. 1,075,114, Brückner et al. (1961)). By one synthesis route, treatment of 17-acetoxy-progesterone with ethyl orthoformate in the presence of an acid catalyst is used to produce the 3-enol ether of the corresponding 3,5-dione. The enol ether is converted to 6-chloro-17α-acetoxyprogesterone by combination with N-chlorosuccinimide, and this chloro compound is dehydrogenated at the 6,7- position to form chlormadinone acetate on treatment with chloranil. Whether this is the synthesis route used for commercial production is not known. Chlormadinone acetate is not produced in the US.

From 1965 until late 1970, when the products were withdrawn from the US market, chlormadinone acetate was used in the US as a component of oral contraceptives, as the progestin in oestrogen-progestin tablets used in sequential therapy. The oestrogen used in the US was mestranol, but elsewhere ethinyloestradiol was used also (Merck & Co., 1968).

Although no data are available on the quantity of chlormadinone acetate consumed in the US for oral contraceptives, according to one source the manufacturer of chlormadinone acetate had sold approximately $2.7 million in bulk form to its US licensee and to several overseas licensees in the fiscal year 1970 (Anon., 1972).

Data on production of chlormadinone acetate in the countries of Western Europe are not available. In 1969, one company was reported to be producing it in the Federal Republic of Germany (Anon., 1969). Although it found widespread use in Europe in earlier years, in 1972 total sales of chlormadinone acetate in hormone and contraceptive specialties in Western Europe were limited to France and are estimated to have been less than 20 kg.

---

[1] Data from Chemical Information Services, Stanford Research Institute, USA

Chlormadinone acetate is approved under certain restrictions by the US Food and Drug Administration for use in cattle feed for the synchronization of oestrus in beef heifers and beef cows (US Code of Federal Regulations, 1973).

2.2 Occurrence

Chlormadinone acetate does not occur in nature.

2.3 Analysis

General methods of analysis are summarized in the section, "General Remarks on the Sex Hormones", p. 43.

3. Biological Data Relevant to the Evaluation of Carcinogenic Risk to Man

3.1 Carcinogenicity and related studies in animals

(a) Oral administration

Mouse: The Committee on Safety of Medicines (1972) coordinated the testing of chlormadinone acetate alone or in combination with mestranol. The drugs were evaluated for carcinogenic activity by incorporation in the diet of one strain of mice for 80 weeks. The doses were identified only as low (2-5 times the human dose), medium (50-150 times) and high (200-400 times). The amounts were not specified. There was no increase in the incidence of tumours in any tissues of male or female CF-LP mice given chlormadinone acetate alone in the diet. When it was combined with mestranol (25:1) there was a 5- to 10-fold increase in the incidence of pituitary tumours, but no increase in tumours of other tissues.

Rudali et al. (1972) administered chlormadinone acetate to groups of 19-46 mice at levels of 0.8 and 8 mg/kg of diet (0.8 and 8 ppm). They estimated the daily intakes as 60 and 600 μg, respectively. At an intake of 60 μg/day, the high incidences of breast cancer in female RIII, C3H and (C3H x RIII)F_1 mice were not significantly affected. Untreated, castrated male (C3H x RIII)F_1 mice had an incidence of 16.4% of breast tumours, which was not significantly changed by administration of chlormadinone acetate (60 μg daily), although the development of post-castration adrenal adenomas was inhibited. Treated female mice did not exhibit vaginal keratinization. At a dosage of 600 μg/day, the latent period for breast tumour development was slightly increased in female mice (from 30 to 36 weeks), but there was no significant change in the incidence or latent period of breast tumours appearing in castrated male (C3H x RIII)F_1 mice (80 versus 82 weeks in controls).

Lutestral (97.5% chlormadinone acetate and 2.5% ethinyloestradiol) fed in the diet at 8 ppm (daily intake, 20-23 μg/mouse) did not alter the breast tumour incidence nor the latent period in intact female RIII, C3H or (C3H x RIII)F_1 mice. In intact male (C3H x RIII)F_1 mice the tumour incidence was increased from 0 to 31.2% (0/76 and 10/32) and in castrated male (C3H x RIII)F_1 mice from 32.8 to 77.8% (20/61 and 23/28), with a decrease in the latent period (Rudali, 1974).

Rat: The Committee on Safety of Medicines (1972) reported no differences in tumour incidence in 75 male or 75 female rats fed chlormadinone acetate in the diet at dosages of 2-5 (low), 50-150 (medium) and 200-400 (high) times the human dose for 104 weeks.

Dog: Nelson et al. (1972) gave 0.25 mg/kg bw chlormadinone acetate daily to 20 female beagle dogs, commencing at 26 to 52 weeks of age. After 104 weeks, 4/20 untreated controls had small (<1.0 cm) nodules in mammary tissue, and similar nodules were palpated in 6 dogs fed chlormadinone acetate. Autopsy of 4 control dogs at this time revealed no abnormal mammary proliferation. A further dog receiving chlormadinone acetate had a mammary nodule measuring 2.5 x 2.0 x 2.0 cm, which at autopsy was found to be a well-encapsulated cystic tumour composed of connective tissue and some epithelial elements and proliferation of myoepithelial tissue. It was classified as a benign, mixed, mammary tumour and was reported to be similar to the nodules found by Vallance & Capel-Edwards (1971) in 2/5 dogs treated for 74 months with high doses of progesterone. Nelson et al. (1972) concluded that the beagle dog is relatively more sensitive to progestins than are women. {See also section, "General Remarks on the Sex Hormones", p. 29.}

Nelson et al. (1973) published a more detailed account of mammary nodules which appeared in 4 dogs after four years of treatment with chlormadinone acetate. Of a total of 22 nodules studied, 12 were diagnosed as nodular hyperplasia, 4 as benign, mixed, mammary tumours and 1 as a mammary adenocarcinoma; the 5 remaining nodules contained no mammary tissue.

3.2 Other relevant biological data

See section, "General Remarks on the Sex Hormones", and pp. 38-40.

3.3 Observations in man

See section, "Oestrogens and Progestins in Relation to Human Cancer", p. 219.

4. Comments on Data Reported and Evaluation[1]

4.1 Animal data

Chlormadinone acetate was tested by the oral route in mice, rats and dogs. In mice it was also tested in combination with oestrogen.

Given alone, it produced no increase in the incidence of tumours in mice or in rats but resulted in mammary tumours in dogs. The significance of the tumours in dogs is discussed in the section, "General Remarks on the Sex Hormones", p. 29.

In combination with mestranol, the incidence of pituitary tumours was increased in mice of both sexes; in combination with ethinyloestradiol, it increased the incidence of mammary tumours in intact and castrated males of one hybrid strain.

4.2 Human data

No case reports or epidemiological studies on chlormadinone acetate alone were available to the Working Group. Epidemiological studies on steroid hormones used in oestrogen-progestin contraceptive preparations have been summarized in the section, "Oestrogens and Progestins in Relation to Human Cancer", p. 223.

---

[1] This section should be read in conjunction with the section, "General Conclusions on Hormones", p. 235.

5. References

Anon. (1969) Chemical Week, May 17, p. 67

Anon. (1972) The Wall Street Transcript, July 17, pp. 29,259-29,261

Brückner, K., Hampel, B. & Johnson, U. (1961) Darstellung und Eigenschaften monohalogenierter 3-Keto-$\Delta^{4,6}$-dien-steroide. Ber. dtsch. chem. Ges., 94, 1225-1240

Committee on Safety of Medicines (1972) Carcinogenicity tests of oral contraceptives, London, HMSO

Merck & Co. (1968) The Merck Index, 8th ed., Rahway, N.J., p. 238

Nelson, L.W., Carlton, W.W. & Weikel, J.H., Jr (1972) Canine mammary neoplasms and progestogens. J. Amer. med. Ass., 219, 1601-1606

Nelson, L.W., Weikel, J.H., Jr & Reno, F.E. (1973) Mammary nodules in dogs during four years' treatment with megestrol acetate or chlormadinone acetate. J. nat. Cancer Inst., 51, 1303-1311

Rudali, G. (1974) Induction of tumors in mice with synthetic sex hormones. Gann Monograph (in press)

Rudali, G., Coezy, E. & Chemama, R. (1972) Mammary carcinogenesis in female and male mice receiving contraceptives or gestagens. J. nat. Cancer Inst., 49, 813-819

US Code of Federal Regulations (1973) Washington DC, US Government Printing Office, 21 CFR 121.238

Vallance, D.K. & Capel-Edwards, K. (1971) Chlormadinone and mammary nodules. Brit. med. J., ii, 221-222

MEDROXYPROGESTERONE ACETATE

1. Chemical and Physical Data

1.1 Synonyms and trade names*

Chem. Abstr. No.: 71-58-9

17-Acetoxy-6α-methylpregn-4-ene-3,20-dione; 17α-acetoxy-6α-methylpregn-4-ene-3,20-dione; 17-acetoxy-6α-methylprogesterone; 17α-acetoxy-6α-methylprogesterone; 17-(acetyloxy)-6-methyl(6α)-pregn-4-ene-3,20-dione; 17-hydroxy-6α-methylpregn-4-ene-3,20-dione acetate; 17-hydroxy-6α-methylpregn-4-ene-3,20-dione 17-acetate; 17α-hydroxy-6α-methylpregn-4-ene-3,20-dione acetate; 17α-hydroxy-6α-methylprogesterone acetate; MAP; 6α-methyl-17α-acetoxy-Δ⁴-pregnene-3,20-dione; 6α-methyl-17α-acetoxy-pregn-4-ene-3,20-dione; 6-methyl-17-acetoxyprogesterone; 6α-methyl-17α-acetoxyprogesterone; 6α-methyl-17α-hydroxyprogesterone acetate; 6α-methyl-4-pregnene-3,20-dion-17α-ol acetate; MPA

Depomedroxyprogesterone acetate; Depo Progevera; Depo-Provera; Farlutal; Farlutal Depot; Farlutin; Gesinol; Gestapuran; Gestapuron; Gestovex; Luteocrin Orale; Lutoral (Farmit); Nogest; Oragest; Perlutex; Protex; Provera; Provest; Repromix; Verafem; Veramix; U 8839

1.2 Chemical formula and molecular weight

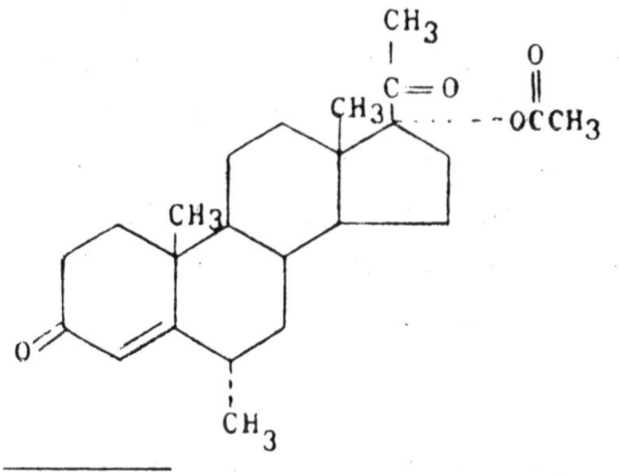

$C_{24}H_{34}O_4$

Mol. wt: 386.5

---

* Trade names include mixtures containing medroxyprogesterone acetate

1.3 Chemical and physical properties of the pure substance

(a) Description: White crystals (from methanol)

(b) Melting-point: 207-209°C

(c) Absorption spectrometry: λ_{max} 240 nm (ϵ = 15900) in ethanol

(d) Refractive index: $\{\alpha\}_D^{25}$ +51° (in dioxane)
     +61° (in chloroform)

(e) Solubility: Practically insoluble in water, soluble at 25°C in ethanol (1 in 800), acetone (1 in 50), chloroform (1 in 10) and dioxane (1 in 60); slightly soluble in ether and methanol

1.4 Technical products and impurities

Medroxyprogesterone acetate is available in the United States as an aqueous suspension in the form of an injection and as tablets (Kastrup, 1973).

2. Production, Use, Occurrence and Analysis

2.1 Production and use[1]

A method for medroxyprogesterone acetate synthesis was first reported by Babcock et al. (1958), and several patents for synthesis routes have since been issued. In one method, the 3,17-ethylene ketal of 17α-hydroxyprogesterone is epoxidized at the 5,6-position with perbenzoic acid, and treatment of the epoxide with methylmagnesium bromide followed by mild acid is used to open the epoxy ring and to methylate the 6-position. The resulting 5α-hydroxy-6-β-methyl-3-one compound is dehydrated to introduce the 4,5-double bond, and the ketal group at the 17-position is removed with acid. Equilibration with a base converts the resulting di-ketone alcohol to the more stable 6α-methyl configuration, and acetylation produces medroxyprogesterone acetate. It is not known whether this is the synthesis route used for commercial production.

---

[1] Data from Chemical Information Services, Stanford Research Institute, USA

No data are available on the quantity of medroxyprogesterone acetate produced by the one US manufacturer.

Medroxyprogesterone acetate in the form of a long-acting injection has been used in human medicine in the US for the treatment of endometriosis, habitual abortion and threatened abortion. However, in October 1973 the US Food and Drug Administration announced plans to withdraw approval for certain strengths and vial sizes of medroxyprogesterone acetate destined for these applications, on the basis of new and old information indicating a lack of substantial evidence that the drug is effective in such treatments and new evidence that it is not safe for use in the treatment of habitual or threatened abortion (US Environmental Protection Agency, 1973).

Medroxyprogesterone acetate is highly active when given orally, thus, in its tablet form, it has been used for the treatment of functional uterine bleeding and secondary amenorrhea, habitual abortion, infertility and threatened abortion. It is also used as an adjunct to cyclic oestrogen therapy, in a test for pregnancy (Kastrup, 1973) and in a palliative treatment for carcinoma of the lining of the uterus (Anon., 1973). However, in October 1973 the US Food and Drug Administration proposed to restrict the approved uses of medroxyprogesterone acetate tablets to the treatment of endometriosis, secondary amenorrhea and of abnormal uterine bleeding due to hormonal imbalance, in the absence of organic pathology such as submucous fibroids or uterine cancer (US Environmental Protection Agency, 1973).

From 1964 until late 1970, when the product was withdrawn from the US market, medroxyprogesterone acetate was used in the US as a component of oral contraceptives, as the progestin in oestrogen-progestin tablets used in combination therapy. The oestrogen used in the US was ethinyloestradiol. The product was removed from the market because studies showed that breast nodules developed in beagles given high doses of medroxyprogesterone acetate.

As of March 1973 medroxyprogesterone acetate injection was reported to be registered as a contraceptive in 38 countries. It was reportedly being used for this purpose in the US (as an injection administered every three months) even though such use had not been approved by the US Food and Drug Administration (Anon., 1973). In October 1973 the US Food and Drug Administration announced plans to permit usage of the medroxyprogesterone acetate injection as a contraceptive for a limited patient population. The manufacturers must provide informational leaflets, there will be certain restrictions on its distribution and provisions for special registration of the practitioners prescribing the drug will be set up under the proposed action (US Environmental Protection Agency, 1973). Prior to these most recent government actions, total US sales of medroxyprogesterone acetate for use in human medicine are estimated to have been less than 500 kg annually.

Data on production of medroxyprogesterone acetate in the countries of Western Europe are not available, but according to one source the injection form of medroxyprogesterone acetate is made only in Belgium and Mexico (Anon., 1973). Total sales of medroxyprogesterone acetate in hormone and contraceptive specialties in Western Europe in 1972 are estimated to have been less than 90 kg. Sales in Italy represented approximately 75% of the total, with lesser amounts sold in The Netherlands, Spain and the United Kingdom.

Medroxyprogesterone acetate is reported to be useful for the prevention of oestrus in bitches (Merck & Co., 1968). It is approved for use in the feed of breeding cattle and ewes for the synchronization of oestrus and ovulation (US Code of Federal Regulations, 1973); however, no data are available on the quantity of medroxyprogesterone acetate consumed in the US for these purposes.

2.2 Occurrence

Medroxyprogesterone acetate does not occur in nature.

2.3 Analysis

General methods of analysis are summarized in the section, "General Remarks on the Sex Hormones", p. 43.

3. Biological Data Relevant to the Evaluation of Carcinogenic Risk to Man

3.1 Carcinogenicity and related studies in animals

(a) Subcutaneous and/or intramuscular injection

In 4 and 16 female beagle dogs administered an i.m. injection of 2.5 mg/kg bw or 62.5 mg/kg bw medroxyprogesterone acetate every 3 months, mammary nodules developed in both groups, the first being detected after 20 and 15 months, respectively. Some mammary nodules also developed in 16 control dogs, the first being detected after 17 months. The difference in the incidence of nodules was not significant; however, there were 10 times as many nodules per dog in the treated groups than in the controls, and, in addition, 3/4 dogs in the higher dosage group had malignant mammary tumours with metastases. All dogs given the higher dose had died or had been killed by the end of the fourth year, and no such malignant tumours were found in dogs that died or were sacrificed prior to month 42 of administration or in any of the control dogs (Finkel & Berliner, 1973; WHO, 1973).

3.2 Other relevant biological data

See section, "General Remarks on the Sex Hormones", and pp. 38-40.

3.3 Observations in man

See section, "Oestrogens and Progestins in Relation to Human Cancer", p. 219.

4. Comments on Data Reported and Evaluation[1]

4.1 Animal data

Medroxyprogesterone acetate was tested by the intramuscular route in dogs and produced malignant mammary tumours. Full details were not available to the Working Group. The significance of the finding in dogs is discussed in the section, "General Remarks on the Sex Hormones", p. 29.

---

[1] This section should be read in conjunction with the section, "General Conclusions on Hormones", p. 235.

4.2 **Human data**

No case reports or epidemiological studies on medroxyprogesterone acetate alone were available to the Working Group. Epidemiological studies on steroid hormones used in oestrogen-progestin contraceptive preparations have been summarized in the section, "Oestrogens and Progestins in Relation to Human Cancer", p. 223.

5. References

Anon. (1973) Chemical & Engineering News, March 5, pp. 10-11

Babcock, J.C., Gutsell, E.S., Herr, M.E., Hogg, J.A., Stucki, J.C., Barnes, L.E. & Dulin, W.E. (1958) 6α-Methyl-17α-hydroxyprogesterone 17-acylates; a new class of potent progestins. J. Amer. chem. Soc., 80, 2904-2905

Finkel, M.J. & Berliner, V.R. (1973) The extrapolation of experimental findings (animals to man): The dilemma of the systemically administered contraceptives. Bull. Soc. pharmacol. environm. Path., 4, 13-18

Kastrup, E.K., ed. (1973) Facts and Comparisons, St. Louis, Missouri, Facts & Comparisons Inc.

Merck & Co. (1968) The Merck Index, 8th ed., Rahway, N.J., p. 648

US Code of Federal Regulations (1973) Washington DC, US Government Printing Office, 21 CFR 121.276

US Environmental Protection Agency (1973) Medroxyprogesterone acetate, injectable contraceptive. US Federal Register, 38, Washington DC, US Government Printing Office, 27940-27942, 27947-27950

WHO (1973) Advances in methods of fertility regulation. Report of a WHO Scientific Group. Wld Hlth Org. techn. Rep. Ser., No. 527, p. 13

19-NORTESTOSTERONE DERIVATIVES

DIMETHISTERONE

1. Chemical and Physical Data

1.1 Synonyms and trade names*

Chem. Abstr. No.: 79-64-1

Dimethylethisterone; 6α,21-dimethylethisterone; 6α,21-dimethyl-17-ethynyl-17β-hydroxyandrost-4-en-3-one; 6α,21-dimethyl-17β-hydroxy-17α-pregn-4-en-20-yn-3-one; 17α-ethynyl-6α,21-dimethyltestosterone; 17α-ethynyl-17-hydroxy-6α,21-dimethylandrost-4-en-3-one; 17β-hydroxy-6α-methyl-17-(1-propynyl)androst-4-en-3-one; 17-hydroxy-6-methyl-17-(1-propynyl)(6α,17β)-androst-4-en-3-one; 17β-hydroxy-6α-methyl-17α-prop-1'-ynyl-androst-4-en-3-one; 6α-methyl-17α-(methylethynyl)testosterone; 6α-methyl-17α-(methylvinyl)testosterone; 6α-methyl-17-(1-propynyl)testosterone; 6α-methyl-17α-propynyltestosterone

Dimethesterone; Oracon; Ovin; Secrodyl; Secrosteron; Tova; Secrovin

1.2 Chemical formula and molecular weight

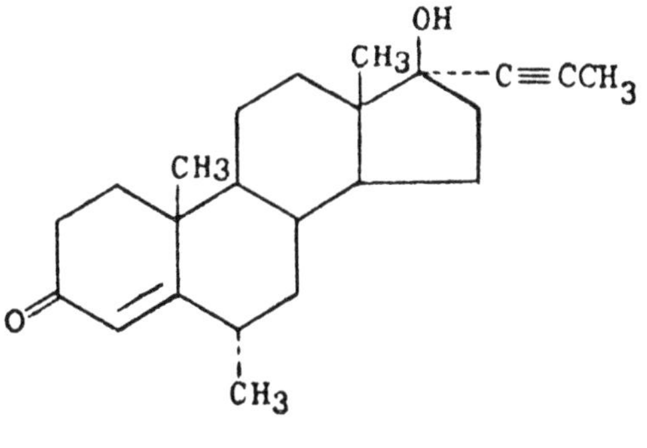

$C_{23}H_{32}O_2$

Mol. wt: 340.5

---

* Trade names include mixtures containing dimethisterone

1.3 Chemical and physical properties of the pure substance

(a) Description: White crystals

(b) Melting-point: 102°C

(c) Absorption spectrometry: λ_{max} 240 nm (ε = 1530) in isopropanol

(d) Optical rotation: $\{\alpha\}_D^{20}$ +10° (1% w/v in chloroform)

(e) Solubility: Practically insoluble in water; soluble at 25°C in 95% ethanol (1 in 3), arachis oil (1 in 80), chloroform (1 in 0.7), pyridine (1 in 1); slightly soluble in acetone

1.4 Technical products and impurities

Dimethisterone is available in the United States only in combination with ethinyloestradiol as tablets for use as oral contraceptives (Kastrup, 1973).

2. Production, Use, Occurrence and Analysis

2.1 Production and use[1]

Synthesis of dimethisterone was first reported in 1959 by Barton et al. (Merck & Co., 1968), and patents were subsequently obtained on several synthesis routes. In one method, dehydroepiandrosterone is treated with potassium acetylide, and the 3- and 17-hydroxyl groups of the resulting 17-ethinyl derivative are then protected as tetrahydropyranyl ethers before introduction of the 21-methyl group with lithium and methyl iodide. After acid-catalyzed removal of the protecting ether groups, the resulting diol is epoxidized at the 5,6-position with perbenzoic acid, and treatment of the epoxide with methylmagnesium bromide followed by mild acid is used to open the epoxy ring and to methylate the 6-position. The resulting 5α-hydroxy-6β-methyl compound is dehydrated to introduce the 4,5-double bond.

---

[1] Data from Chemical Information Services, Stanford Research Institute, USA

Equilibration with a base produces dimethisterone, which has the more stable 6α-methyl configuration. Whether this is the synthesis route used for commercial production is not known. Dimethisterone is not produced in the US.

Dimethisterone has been used in the US as a component of oral contraceptives since 1965, as the progestin in oestrogen-progestin tablets used in sequential therapy. The oestrogen used in the US is ethinyloestradiol (Merck & Co., 1968). Total US sales of dimethisterone for use in oral contraceptives are estimated to be less than 600 kg annually.

Data on production of dimethisterone in the countries of Western Europe are not available, but it is believed that one company in the UK manufactures the chemical. Total sales of dimethisterone in hormone and contraceptive specialties in Western Europe in 1972 were limited to the UK and are estimated to have been less than 10 kg. Dimethisterone has also been used in the UK in conjunction with ethinyloestradiol for early diagnosis of pregnancy and for the treatment of secondary amenorrhea of short duration, of endometriosis and of genital hypoplasia (Blacow, 1972).

2.2 Occurrence

Dimethisterone does not occur in nature.

2.3 Analysis

General methods of analysis are summarized in the section, "General Remarks on the Sex Hormones", p. 43.

3. Biological Data Relevant to the Evaluation of Carcinogenic Risk to Man

3.1 Carcinogenicity and related studies in animals

No data were available to the Working Group.

3.2 Other relevant biological data

See section, "General Remarks on the Sex Hormones", and pp. 38-40.

3.3 Observations in man

See section, "Oestrogens and Progestins in Relation to Human Cancer", p. 219.

4. Comments on Data Reported and Evaluation[1]

4.1 Animal data

No data were available to the Working Group.

4.2 Human data

No case reports or epidemiological studies were available to the Working Group. Epidemiological studies on steroid hormones used in oestrogen-progestin oral contraceptive preparations have been summarized in the section, "Oestrogens and Progestins in Relation to Human Cancer", p. 223.

---

[1] This section should be read in conjunction with the section "General Conclusions on Hormones", p. 235.

5. References

Blacow, N.W., ed. (1972) *Martindale. The Extra Pharmacopoeia*, 26th ed., London, The Pharmaceutical Press

Kastrup, E.D., ed. (1973) *Facts and Comparisons*, St. Louis, Missouri, Facts & Comparisons Inc.

Merck & Co. (1968) *The Merck Index*, 8th ed., Rahway, N.J., p. 373

ETHYNODIOL DIACETATE

1. Chemical and Physical Data

1.1 Synonyms and trade names*

Chem. Abstr. No.: 29-77-67

3β,17β-Diacetoxy-17α-ethynyl-4-estrene; 3β,17α-diacetoxy-19-nor-17α-pregn-4-en-20-yne; ethynodiol acetate; 17α-ethynyl-3,17-dihydroxy-4-estrene diacetate; 17α-ethynylestr-4-ene-3β,17β-diol diacetate; 17α-ethynyl-4-estrene-3β,17β-diol diacetate; 17α-ethynyl-Δ⁴-estrene-3β,17β-diol diacetate; 17α-ethynyl-4-estrene-3β,17-diol diacetate; 17α-ethynyl-19-norandrost-4-ene-3β,17β-diol diacetate; 19-nor-17α-pregn-4-en-20-yne-3β,17-diol diacetate; (3β,17α)-19-norpregn-4-en-20-yne-3,17-diol diacetate

Demulen; Demulen 50; Femulen; FH 027; Lueolas; Luteonorm; Luto-Metrodiol; Metrodiol Diacetate; Metrulen; Metrulene; Metrulen M; Neovulen; Ovulen; Ovulen 0.5; Ovulen 1.0; Ovulen 1/50; Ovulen 50; Ovulene 50; Ovulen Mite; SC 11800

1.2 Chemical formula and molecular weight

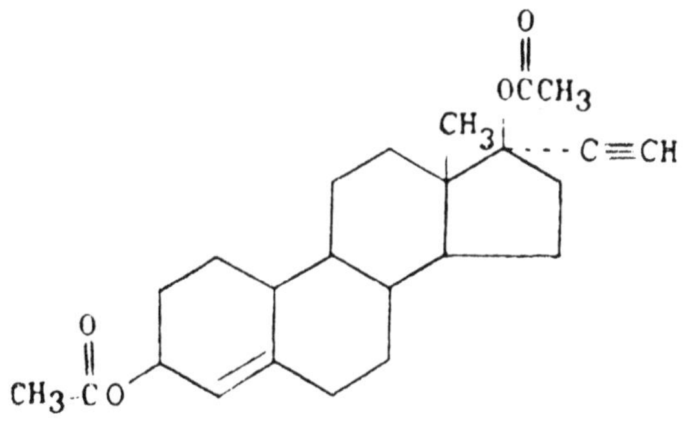

$C_{24}H_{32}O_4$

Mol. wt: 384.5

---

* Trade names include mixtures containing ethynodiol diacetate

1.3 **Chemical and physical properties of the pure substance**

(a) Description: White crystals (from methanol and water)

(b) Melting-point: 126-127°C

(c) Optical rotation: $\{\alpha\}_D^{20}$ -72.5° (in chloroform)

(d) Solubility: Practically insoluble in water; soluble at 25°C in 95% ethanol (1 in 15), chloroform (1 in 1), ether (1 in 3.5), acetone and oils

1.4 **Technical products and impurities**

Ethynodiol diacetate is available in the United States only in combination with mestranol or ethinyloestradiol as tablets for use as oral contraceptives (Kastrup, 1973).

2. Production, Use, Occurrence and Analysis

2.1 **Production and use**[1]

A method for the synthesis of ethynodiol diacetate was first patented in the US in 1965 (US 3,176,013, granted to P.D. Klimstra (Merck & Co., 1968)). In this method, norethindrone is reduced (using a solution of the product of the reaction of tert-butyl alcohol with lithium aluminium hydride) to ethynodiol, and this is acetylated with acetic anhydride in pyridine to produce ethynodiol diacetate. Whether this is the synthesis route used for commercial production is not known. Ethynodiol diacetate is not produced in the US.

Ethynodiol diacetate has been used in the US as a component of oral contraceptives since 1966, as the progestin in oestrogen-progestin tablets used in combination therapy. The oestrogen used in the US is mestranol or ethinyloestradiol (Kastrup, 1973). Total US sales of ethynodiol diacetate for use in oral contraceptives are estimated to be less than 400 kg annually.

---

[1] Data from Chemical Information Services, Stanford Research Institute, USA

Data on production of ethynodiol diacetate in the countries of Western Europe are not available, but production and sales are believed to be concentrated in a small number of companies. Total sales of ethynodiol diacetate in hormone and contraceptive specialties in Western Europe in 1972 are estimated to have been less than 75 kg. Sales in the UK represented approximately 50% of the total, with lesser amounts sold in France, Italy and The Netherlands. In addition to its use as a component of oral contraceptives, ethynodiol diacetate has been used in Western Europe in combination with mestranol for the treatment of various disorders of menstruation, fertility and pregnancy (Blacow, 1972).

2.2 Occurrence

Ethynodiol diacetate does not occur in nature.

2.3 Analysis

General methods of analysis are summarized in the section, "General Remarks on the Sex Hormones", p. 43.

3. Biological Data Relevant to the Evaluation of Carcinogenic Risk to Man

3.1 Carcinogenicity and related studies in animals

(a) Oral administration

Mouse: The Committee on Safety of Medicines (1972) coordinated a trial of ethynodiol diacetate alone or in combination with oestrogens. The drugs were evaluated for carcinogenic activity by incorporation in the diet of one strain of mice for 80 weeks. The doses were identified only as low (2-5 times the human dose), medium (50-150 times) and high (200-400 times). The amounts were not specified. Ethynodiol diacetate alone did not increase the incidence of tumours in any tissues of treated CF-LP mice compared with controls. When ethynodiol diacetate was administered in combination with mestranol (1:1, 10:1 and 20:1), the incidences of pituitary tumours in groups of 120 males and 120 females for each combination were 2-8 in male and female controls and 23-37 in treated groups. Ethynodiol diacetate in combination with ethinyloestradiol in proportions of 2:1 and 20:1 increased the incidences of pituitary tumours to 30-94 per group of 120 animals.

Rudali et al. (1972) showed that ethynodiol diacetate (0.68 mg/kg bw/day) given to castrated male (C3H x RIII)F_1 mice increased mammary tumour incidence from 16 to 46% but did not affect the latency period (81 versus 82 weeks). In intact (C3H x RIII)F_1 females administered 0.56-0.75 or 75-10(µg/kg bw/day, neither mammary tumour incidence nor latent period were affected.

Ovulen (90% ethynodiol diacetate and 10% mestranol) mixed in the diet at 3 ppm (intake, 7.5-10 µg/mouse/day) increased the incidence of breast tumours in intact male (C3H x RIII)F_1 mice from 0 to 56% (0/76 and 14/25) and in castrated males from 16 to 75% (10/61 and 21/28). The high incidence (96-98%) and short latent period of tumour induction (30-33 weeks) were not altered in intact females. In ovariectomized females the tumour incidence was not altered (82 and 77%) by Ovulen; but the latent period was reduced in both ovariectomized females (from 49 weeks to 26 weeks) and castrated males (from 82 weeks to 43 weeks) (Rudali, 1974).

Rat: The Committee on Safety of Medicines (1972) reported no increase in incidences of tumours in groups of 105-180 rats fed ethynodiol diacetate alone or with mestranol (10:1) at doses of 2-5 (low), 50-150 (medium) or 200-400 (high) times the human dose. In male rats treated with ethynodiol diacetate alone, benign mammary tumours occurred in 10% of treated rats compared with 0% in controls, and malignant mammary tumours occurred in 5% of treated rats compared with 3% in controls. In combination with ethinyl-oestradiol (2:1), there were malignant mammary tumours in 10% of treated males compared with 0% in controls, and the incidence of malignant mammary tumours was increased in female rats administered the combination from 5% in controls to 14%. Ethynodiol diacetate with mestranol (20:1) increased the incidence of malignant mammary tumours in one group of 120 female rats from 0 to 15%; the same treatment in a group of 120 males increased the incidence from 3 to 7%. In a further group of 105 female rats receiving ethynodiol diacetate plus mestranol (20:1) the incidence of malignant mammary tumours was not increased (3% in controls, compared with 0% in treated rats).

3.2 Other relevant biological data

See section, "General Remarks on the Sex Hormones", and pp. 38-40.

3.3 Observations in man

See section, "Oestrogens and Progestins in Relation to Human Cancer", p. 219.

4. Comments on Data Reported and Evaluation[1]

4.1 Animal data

Ethynodiol diacetate was tested alone or in combination with oestrogens by the oral route in mice and rats. Given alone, it did not increase the incidence of tumours in female mice or female rats; in castrated male mice it increased the incidence of mammary tumours, and in male rats it produced benign mammary tumours. In combination with oestrogens it increased the incidence of malignant mammary tumours in some groups of male and female rats.

4.2 Human data

No case reports or epidemiological studies on ethynodiol diacetate alone were available to the Working Group. Epidemiological studies on steroid hormones used in oestrogen-progestin contraceptive preparations have been summarized in the section, "Oestrogens and Progestins in Relation to Human Cancer", p. 223.

---

[1] This section should be read in conjuction with the section "General Conclusions on Hormones", p. 235.

5. References

Blacow, N.W., ed. (1972) Martindale. The Extra Pharmacopoeia, 26th ed., London, The Pharmaceutical Press

Committee on Safety of Medicines (1972) Carcinogenicity tests of oral contraceptives, London, HMSO

Kastrup, E.K., ed. (1973) Facts and Comparisons, St. Louis, Missouri, Facts & Comparisons Inc.

Merck & Co. (1968) The Merck Index, 8th ed., Rahway, N.J., p. 442

Rudali, G. (1974) Induction of tumors in mice with synthetic sex hormones. Gann Monogr. (in press)

Rudali, G., Coezy, E. & Chemama, R. (1972) Mammary carcinogenesis in female and male mice receiving contraceptives or gestagens. J. nat. Cancer Inst., 49, 813-819

NORETHISTERONE AND NORETHISTERONE ACETATE

1. Chemical and Physical Data

Norethisterone

1.1 Synonyms and trade names*

Chem. Abstr. No.: 68-22-4

Anhydrohydroxynorprogesterone; 17α-ethinylestr-4-en-17β-ol-3-one; 17α-ethinyl-17β-hydroxy-Δ^4-estren-3-one; ethinylnortestosterone; 17α-ethinyl-19-nortestosterone; 17α-ethynyl-4-estren-17-ol-3-one; 17α-ethynyl-17-hydroxy-4-estren-3-one; 17α-ethynyl-17β-hydroxyestr-4-en-3-one; 17α-ethynyl-17β-hydroxy-19-norandrost-4-en-3-one; 17α-ethynyl-19-norandrost-4-en-17β-ol-3-one; 17α-ethynyl-19-nor-4-androsten-17β-ol-3-one; 17α-ethynyl-19-nortestosterone; 17-ethynyl-19-nortestosterone; 17-hydroxy-19-nor-17α-pregn-4-en-20-yn-3-one; 17-hydroxy(17α)-19-norpregn-4-en-20-yn-3-one; 17β-hydroxy-19-norpregn-4-en-20-yn-3-one; norethindrone; 19-norethindrone; norethisteron; 19-norethisterone; norethyndron; norethynodrone; 19-nor-17α-ethynylandrosten-17β-ol-3-one; 19-nor-17α-ethynyl-17β-hydroxy-4-androsten-3-one; 19-nor-17α-ethynyltestosterone; norpregneninlone

Anovlar 21; Anovule; Anzolan; Conlumin; Conlunett; Conlunett 21; Conlutan; Conluten; Dianor; Gynostat; Gynovlar; Nor 50; Norfor; Noriday; Noridei; Norinyl; Norinyl 1; Norinyl 2; Norluten; Norlutin; Norluton; Nor-QD; Norquentiel; NSC-9564; Orlestrin; Orthonovin; Ortho-Novin; Ortho-Novin 2; Ortho-Novin 1/50; Ortho-Novin 1/80; Ortho-Novin Mite; Ortho-Novin Sq.; Orthonovum; Orthonovum N; Ortho-Novum; Ortho-Novum 1/50; Ortho-Novum 1/80; Ortho-Novum 2; Ortho-Novum Sq.; Plan; Primolutin; Primolut N; Primosiston; Progynon C; Regovar

---

* Trade names include mixtures containing norethisterone

1.2 Chemical formula and molecular weight

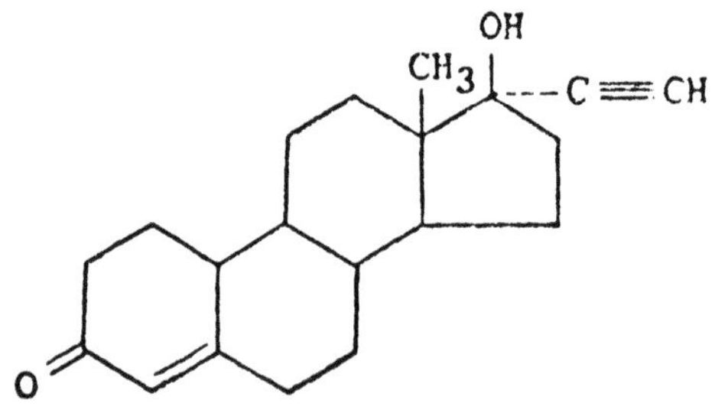

$C_{20}H_{26}O_2$

Mol. wt: 298.4

1.3 Chemical and physical properties of the pure substance

(a) Description: White crystals (from ethyl acetate)

(b) Melting-point: 203-204°C

(c) Absorption spectrometry: λ_{max} 240 nm (ε = 17 380) in ethanol

(d) Optical rotation: $\{\alpha\}_D^{20}$ -31.7° (in chloroform)

(e) Solubility: Practically insoluble in water; soluble at 25°C in 95% ethanol (1 in 150), acetone (1 in 80), chloroform (1 in 30) and pyridine (1 in 5); slightly soluble in vegetable oils

1.4 Technical products and impurities

Norethisterone is available in the United States in the form of tablets containing only norethisterone and of tablets containing combinations of norethisterone with mestranol (Kastrup, 1973).

Norethisterone acetate

1.1 Synonyms and trade names*

Chem. Abstr. No.: 51-98-9

17-Acetoxy-19-nor-17α-pregn-4-en-20-yn-3-one; 17β-acetoxy-19-nor-17α-pregn-4-en-20-yn-3-one; 17-acetyloxy(17α)-19-norpregn-4-estren-17β-ol-acetate-3-one; 17-ENT; ENTA; 17α-ethinyl-19-nortestosterone

---

* Trade names include mixtures containing norethisterone acetate

acetate; 17α-ethinyl-19-nortestosterone-17β-acetate; 17α-ethynyl-17β-acetoxy-19-norandrost-4-en-3-one; 17α-ethynyl-17-hydroxyestr-4-en-3-one acetate; 17α-ethynyl-19-nortestosterone acetate; 17-hydroxy-19-nor-17α-pregn-4-en-20-yn-3-one acetate; 17β-hydroxy-19-nor-17α-pregn-4-en-20-yn-3-one acetate; norethindrone acetate; norethisteron acetate; norethynyltestosterone acetate; 19-norethynyl-testosterone acetate; norethysterone acetate

Ablacton; Anovlar; Anovlar 21; Controvlar; Duogynon Oral; Etalontin; Gestest; Gynovlane; Milli-Anovlar; Minovlar; N Gestakliman; Norinyl; Norlestrin; Norlutate; Norlutate A; Norlutin acetate; Orlest 28; Primodos; Primolut-Nor; Primosiston; Profinix; Progylut; Prolestrin

1.2 <u>Chemical formula and molecular weight</u>

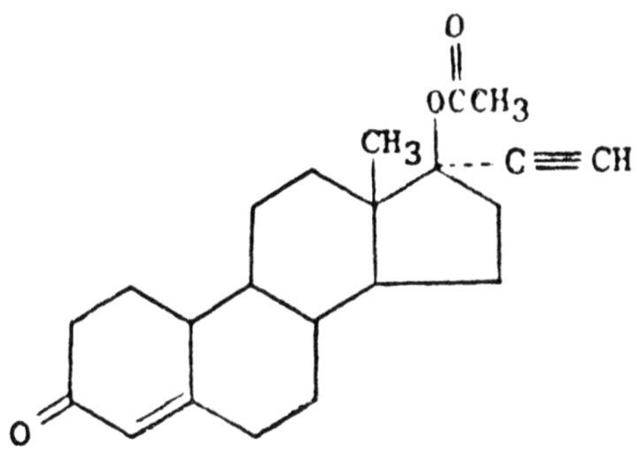

$C_{22}H_{28}O_3$

Mol. wt: 340.5

1.3 <u>Chemical and physical properties of the pure substance</u>

(<u>a</u>) <u>Description</u>: White crystals (from methylene chloride and hexane)

(<u>b</u>) <u>Melting-point</u>: 161-162°C

(<u>c</u>) <u>Absorption spectrometry</u>: λ_{max} 240 nm (ε = 18690)

(<u>d</u>) <u>Solubility</u>: Practically insoluble in water; soluble at 25°C in 95% ethanol (1 in 12.5) and acetone (1 in 4); also soluble in chloroform, dioxane and ether

1.4 Technical products and impurities

Norethisterone acetate is available in the United States in the form of tablets containing only norethisterone acetate and of tablets containing combinations of norethisterone acetate with ethinyloestradiol (Kastrup, 1973).

2. Production, Use, Occurrence and Analysis

Norethisterone

2.1 Production and use[1]

Synthesis of norethisterone was first reported in 1954 by Djerassi et al. (Merck & Co., 1968), and several patents were subsequently obtained. In one method, oestrone (derived from diosgenin) is converted to its methyl ether, which is first reduced to oestradiol 3-methyl ether with lithium aluminium hydride and then further reduced by a Birch reduction to give the 1,4-dihydroaromatic compound. Oppenauer oxidation produces the 17-ketone, which is ethynylated with acetylene to produce the 17-ethynyl carbinol. Subsequent acid hydrolysis of the 3-methyl ether using a mineral acid such as hydrochloric acid produces norethisterone. Whether this is the synthesis route used for commercial production is not known.

Norethisterone is not produced in the US, although since 1957 small quantities have been used in human medicine as orally-active progestin for the treatment of such conditions as amenorrhea and endometriosis. Norethisterone has been widely used in the US since 1962 as the progestin in progestin-oestrogen combination therapy oral contraceptive products, and since 1966 as the progestin in the progestin-oestrogen tablets used in conjunction with oestrogen tablets in sequential therapy. The oestrogen used in the US is mestranol.

One source has estimated that one of the marketers of these oral contraceptive products purchased bulk norethisterone valued at $10 million

---

[1] Data from Chemical Information Services, Stanford Research Institute, USA

in the fiscal year 1971; it was also estimated that these purchases would increase to $12-13 million in 1972 (Anon., 1972).

In late 1972, the US Food and Drug Administration approved the use of new, oestrogen-free oral contraceptives. Such products contain only a progestin, norethisterone, and are available as "mini-pills" which are administered on a continuous daily dosage throughout the year (US Food and Drug Administration, 1972). Thus, although total US sales of norethisterone for use in human medicine are estimated to have been less than 2 000 kg annually prior to the approval of these "mini-pills", this usage may have grown considerably in the past year - not only because of the FDA approval but also because of the expiration of the US patent on norethisterone in May 1973.

Norethisterone is also used as an intermediate (although probably not isolated) in the commercial synthesis of norethisterone acetate and possibly in the synthesis of ethynodiol diacetate.

Data on production of norethisterone in the countries of Western Europe are not available, but it is believed that one company in the Federal Republic of Germany manufactures the chemical. Total sales of norethisterone in hormone and contraceptive specialties in Western Europe in 1972 are estimated to have been less than 325 kg. Sales in France represented approximately 45% of the total, with lesser amounts sold in the Federal Republic of Germany, the United Kingdom and The Netherlands.

One source has indicated that the basic manufacturer of norethisterone processes barbasco roots in Mexico to obtain diosgenin and then makes intermediates which are converted into the finished, bulk norethisterone in Freeport, Grand Bahamas (Anon., 1972).

2.2 Occurrence

Norethisterone does not occur in nature.

2.3 Analysis

General methods of analysis are summarized in the section, "General Remarks on the Sex Hormones", p. 43.

Norethisterone acetate

2.1 Production and use[1]

Methods for norethisterone acetate synthesis were first patented in the US in 1960 (US 2,964,537). In one method, acetic anhydride and pyridine are used for the acetylation of norethisterone.

Norethisterone acetate is not produced in the US, although it is used in human medicine as an orally-active progestin (twice as potent as norethisterone) for the treatment of amenorrhea and endometriosis. It is also used in combination with ethinyloestradiol in a test for pregnancy. The quantity of norethisterone acetate used for these purposes is believed to be significantly less than the quantity used in oral contraceptives.

Norethisterone acetate has been used in the US since 1964 as the progestin in progestin-oestrogen combination therapy oral contraceptive products (the oestrogen used in the US is ethinyloestradiol). One source has estimated that the US marketer of these oral contraceptive products purchased bulk norethisterone acetate valued at $5-6 million in fiscal 1971 and $7-8 million in 1972 (Anon., 1972). Total US sales of norethisterone acetate for use in human medicine are estimated to be less than 100 kg annually.

Norethisterone acetate is reportedly produced in Freeport, Grand Bahamas, from diosgenin-derived intermediates imported from Mexico (Anon., 1972).

Data on production of norethisterone acetate in the countries of Western Europe are not available, but it is believed to be manufactured by one company in the Federal Republic of Germany. In addition to its use as a component of oral contraceptives, norethisterone acetate has been used in Western Europe in combination with ethinyloestradiol for the treatment of dysmenorrhea, endometriosis, subfertility, for medically indicated contraception and for early diagnosis of pregnancy (Blacow, 1972).

---

[1] Data from Chemical Information Services, Stanford Research Institute, USA

2.2 Occurrence

Norethisterone acetate does not occur in nature.

2.3 Analysis

General methods of analysis are summarized in the section, "General Remarks on the Sex Hormones", p. 43.

3. Biological Data Relevant to the Evaluation of Carcinogenic Risk to Man

3.1 Carcinogenicity and related studies in animals

(a) Oral administration

Mouse: Poel (1966) administered a mixture of norethisterone and ethinyloestradiol (50:1) to female C57L mice by gavage at dosages of 7 and 70 µg in peanut oil 5 times per week. Pituitary tumours were found at autopsy in 5/8 mice on the higher dose and in 7/15 on the lower dose, after 84-89 weeks, compared with 2/15 controls. Hepatomas were found in 10/96 of the initial groups of mice used in this and in a concurrent experiment with norethynodrel plus mestranol, but there is no indication in which groups they arose. No hepatomas were found in 48 control mice.

The Committee on Safety of Medicines (1972) coordinated a trial of norethisterone and its acetate alone or in combination with oestrogens. The drugs were evaluated for carcinogenic activity by incorporation into the diet of one strain of mice, the doses being identified only as low (2-5 times the human dose), medium (50-150 times) and high (200-400 times). The amounts were not specified. An increased incidence of benign liver-cell tumours occurred in groups of male CF-LP mice with both norethisterone and its acetate (33 and 35 out of 120 compared to 18 and 19 in the 2 groups of 120 controls). Treated female CF-LP mice did not show an increase in liver-cell tumour incidence. Incidences of pituitary tumours were increased in female mice fed norethisterone alone (from 4-8/120 in controls to 23/120 in treated mice), and in groups of male and female mice given combinations of norethisterone acetate with ethinyloestradiol (50:1) (from 2/120 to 25/120 in males and from 4-8/120 to 32/120 in females) or of norethisterone plus mestranol (20:1) (2/120 to 15/120 in males and 4-8/120 to 31/120 in females). Norethisterone acetate did not increase the incidence of pituitary tumours when fed alone.

Rat: The Committee on Safety of Medicines (1972) (for details see under "mouse") reported increases in the numbers of benign liver-cell tumours in groups of 120 male but not in female rats fed norethisterone or norethisterone plus mestranol (20:1) (12% and 23% versus 4% in controls). The same treatments induced benign and malignant mammary tumours in male rats (4% and 12% compared with 0% in controls). Norethisterone plus mestranol increased the incidence of malignant mammary tumours in females from 5 to 30%. Feeding of norethisterone acetate plus ethinyloestradiol (50:1) was associated with an increase in the incidence of benign mammary tumours in male rats from 2 to 28%, but there were no increases in the incidences of tumours of other tissues in either males or females with this regimen.

In groups of 100 male and 100 female controls and of 50 male and 50 female test Sprague-Dawley rats fed 75 ppm of a mixture of 98% norethisterone acetate and 2% ethinyloestradiol in the diet, an increase in the incidences of regenerative liver nodules (10% versus 2%) and of liver adenomas (4% versus 0%) was observed. The incidence of benign mammary tumours was unchanged, but the proportions of fibroepithelial tumours to adenomas varied from 57% and 5% in controls to 38% and 32% in the test groups. In males the proportions were 1% and 0% in controls and 36% and 2% in the test groups. With a dietary concentration of the mixture of 7.5 ppm the incidence of regenerative liver nodules was still increased (13% versus 2% in the controls) as was that of liver adenomas (3% versus 0%). The incidence of benign mammary tumours was unchanged, and the proportions of fibroepithelial tumours to adenomas were similar in male and female controls and in test groups. The incidence of adenocarcinomas was slightly increased only in the test groups on a 75 ppm mixture (8% versus 2% in controls) (Schardein et al., 1970).

Pretreatment of intact female Sprague-Dawley rats with 0.25 mg Norlestrin (norethisterone plus ethinyloestradiol, 50:1) daily for 10 days increased the incidence of breast tumours induced by a single oral administration of 8 mg DMBA from 45% to 81% in groups of 38 and 22 rats. Pretreatment with 1 mg Norlestrin for 10 days did not significantly increase the incidence of such tumours produced by DMBA (McCarthy, 1965).

(b) Subcutaneous implantation

Mouse: Lipschütz et al. (1966, 1967) reported so-called granulosa-cell tumours of the ovaries in 13/25 BALB/c mice implanted with pellets containing 40% norethisterone and 60% cholesterol for 76-77 weeks. Only 2 of these were macroscopic in size. The absorption of norethisterone was estimated to be between 3.6 and 15.9 µg/day.

3.2 Other relevant biological data

See section, "General Remarks on the Sex Hormones", and pp. 38-40.

3.3 Observations in man

See section, "Oestrogens and Progestins in Relation to Human Cancer", p. 219.

4. Comments on Data Reported and Evaluation[1]

4.1 Animal data

Norethisterone or its acetate were tested in mice by oral administration and by subcutaneous implantation and in rats by oral administration. When administered alone to mice norethisterone increased the incidence of benign liver-cell tumours in males, of pituitary tumours in females and produced a low incidence of microscopic ovarian tumours in females. The acetate alone only increased the incidence of benign liver-cell tumours in males.

Norethisterone in combination with mestranol, or the acetate in combination with ethinyloestradiol, increased the incidence of pituitary tumours in both sexes. In addition, norethisterone in combination with ethinyloestradiol increased the incidence of pituitary tumours in female mice.

---

[1] This section should be read in conjunction with the section, "General Conclusions on Hormones", p. 235.

In rats, norethisterone alone increased the incidence of benign liver-cell tumours in males. In combination with mestranol it increased the incidence of benign liver-cell tumours in males and of malignant mammary tumours in both sexes. Norethisterone acetate in combination with ethinyloestradiol increased the incidence of benign mammary tumours in males in one study and increased the incidence of benign liver-cell and mammary tumours in both sexes in a further study.

4.2 Human data

No case reports or epidemiological studies on norethisterone or its acetate alone were available. Epidemiological studies on steroid hormones used in oestrogen-progestin contraceptive preparations have been summarized in the section, "Oestrogens and Progestins in Relation to Human Cancer", p. 223.

5. References

Anon. (1972) The Wall Street Transcript, July 17, pp. 29,259-29,261

Blacow, N.W., ed. (1972) Martindale. The Extra Pharmacopoeia, 26th ed., London, The Pharmaceutical Press

Committee on the Safety of Medicines (1972) Carcinogenicity tests of oral contraceptives, London, HMSO

Kastrup, E.K., ed. (1973) Facts and Comparisons, St. Louis, Missouri, Facts & Comparisons Inc.

Lipschütz, A., Iglesias, R., Salinas, S. & Panasevich, V.I. (1966) Experimental conditions under which contraceptive steroids may become toxic. Nature (Lond.), 212, 686-688

Lipschütz, A., Iglesias, R., Panasevich, V.I. & Salinas, S. (1967) Ovarian tumours and other ovarian changes induced in mice by two 19-nor-contraceptives. Brit. J. Cancer, 21, 153-159

McCarthy, J.D. (1965) Influence of two contraceptives on induction of mammary cancer in rats. Amer. J. Surg., 110, 720-723

Merck & Co. (1968) The Merck Index, 8th ed., Rahway, N.J., p. 748

Poel, W.E. (1966) Pituitary tumours in mice after prolonged feeding of synthetic progestins. Science, 154, 402-403

Schardein, J.L., Kaump, D.H., Woosley, E.T. & Jellema, M.M. (1970) Long-term toxicologic and tumorigenesis studies on an oral contraceptive agent in albino rats. Toxicol. appl. Pharmacol., 16, 10-23

US Food and Drug Administration (1972) FDA Drug Bulletin, December, Washington DC, US Government Printing Office

NORETHYNODREL

1. Chemical and Physical Data

1.1 Synonyms and trade names*

Chem. Abstr. No.: 68-23-5

17α-Ethinyl-5,10-estrenolone; 17α-ethinyl-17β-hydroxy-$\Delta^{5(10)}$-estren-3-one; 17α-ethynyl-5(10)-estren-17-ol-3-one; 17α-ethynylestr-5(10)-en-17β-ol-3-one; 17α-ethynylestr-5(10)-en-17β-ol-3-one; 17α-ethynyl-17-hydroxy-5(10)-estren-3-one; 17α-ethynyl-17β-hydroxy-$\Delta^{5(10)}$-estren-3-one; 17α-ethynyl-17β-hydroxyestr-5(10)-en-3-one; 17α-ethynyl-17β-hydroxy-3-oxo-$\Delta^{5(10)}$-estrene; 17α-ethynyl-19-nor-5(10)-androsten-17β-ol-3-one; 17-hydroxy-19-nor-17α-pregn-5(10)-en-20-yn-3-one; 17-hydroxy(17α)-19-norpregn-5(10)-en-20-yn-3-one; 13-methyl-17-ethynyl-17-hydroxy-1,2,3,4,6,7,8,9,11,12,13,14,16,17-tetradecahydro-15H-cyclopenta{a}phananthren-3-one; norethinynodrel; norethynodral; 19-norethynodrel

Conovid; Conovid E; Enavid; Enavid E; Enidrel; Enovid; Enovid E; Noretynodrel; Norolen; Orgametril; Previson; Singestol

1.2 Chemical formula and molecular weight

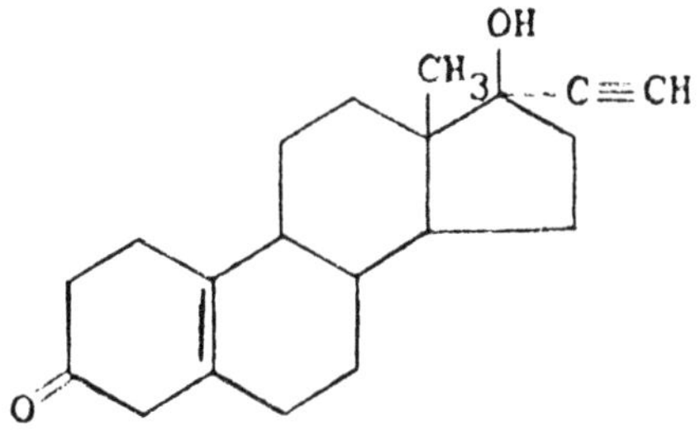

$C_{20}H_{26}O_2$
Mol. wt: 298.4

---

* Trade names include mixtures containing norethynodrel

1.3 Chemical and physical properties of the pure substance

(a) Description: White crystals (from aqueous methanol)

(b) Melting-point: 169-170°C

(c) Optical rotation: $\{\alpha\}_D^{25}$ +108° (1% w/v in chloroform)

(d) Solubility: Practically insoluble in water; soluble at 25°C in 95% ethanol (1 in 30), chloroform (1 in 7) and ether (1 in 60); also soluble in acetone and methanol

1.4 Technical products and impurities

Norethynodrel is available in the United States in the form of tablets containing only norethynodrel and of tablets containing combinations of norethynodrel with mestranol (Kastrup, 1973). Norethynodrel as normally manufactured has been reported to contain up to 1.5% of mestranol (Blacow, 1972).

2. Production, Use, Occurrence and Analysis

2.1 Production and use[1]

Methods for norethynodrel synthesis were first patented in the US in 1954 and 1955 (US patents 2,691,028 and 2,725,389, granted to F.B. Colton). By one synthesis route, oestrone (derived from diosgenin) is converted to its methyl ether, which is first reduced to oestradiol 3-methyl ether with lithium aluminium hydride and then further reduced by a Birch reduction to give the 1,4-dihydroaromatic compound. Oppenauer oxidation produces the 17-ketone, which is ethynylated with acetylene to produce the 17-ethynyl carbinol. Subsequent acid hydrolysis of the 3-methyl ether using a weak acid such as oxalic acid produces norethynodrel. Whether this is the synthesis route used for commercial production is not known. Norethynodrel is not produced in the US.

---

[1] Data from Chemical Information Services, Stanford Research Institute, USA

Norethynodrel is used in human medicine only in combinations with the oestrogen, mestranol. Such combinations are used for the treatment of endometriosis and hypermenorrhea, but the quantity of norethynodrel used for such treatments is believed to be quite small compared to the quantity used in oral contraceptives.

Norethynodrel has been used in the US since 1961 as the progestin in progestin-oestrogen combination therapy oral contraceptive products (the oestrogen used in the US is mestranol). Total US sales or norethynodrel for use in human medicine are estimated to be less than 400 kg annually.

Data on production of norethynodrel in the countries of Western Europe are not available but production and sales are believed to be concentrated in a small number of companies. Total sales of norethynodrel in hormone and contraceptive specialties in Western Europe in 1972 are estimated to have been less than 10 kg. Sales in the UK represented approximately 80% of the total, with lesser amounts sold in Italy.

2.2 Occurrence

Norethynodrel does not occur in nature.

2.3 Analysis

General methods of analysis are given in the section, "General Remarks on the Sex Hormones", p. 43.

3. Biological Data Relevant to the Evaluation of Carcinogenic Risk to Man

3.1 Carcinogenicity and related studies in animals

In some of the following investigations norethynodrel was administered as the commercial product "Enovid", containing 98.5% norethynodrel and 1.5% mestranol. The experimental data has been summarized below and also under "mestranol". Thus, the results of such treatment may reflect the activity of either constituent or of the combination.

(a) Oral administration

Mouse: Poel (1966) reported the appearance of pituitary tumours in female C57L mice given 7 or 70 µg of a mixture of norethynodrel plus mestranol (50:1) in oil 5 times per week by gavage. At the higher dose level, 7/7 mice had pituitary tumours after 84 weeks, as did 6/11 on the lower dose, compared with 2/15 controls. Hepatomas were found in 10/96 of the initial group of the C57L mice used in this and in a concurrent experiment with norethisterone and ethinyloestradiol, but there is no indication in the report in which group they arose. No hepatomas were found in 48 control animals.

Dunn (1969) fed a liquid diet (Metrecal) containing Enovid to female BALB/c mice and estimated that each mouse consumed 10-12.5 µg of the drug each day. All of the 8 mice surviving more than 74 weeks of treatment had early or infiltrating carcinomas of the cervix. No carcinomas of the uterus, cervix or vagina were found in 44 untreated females surviving 103-129 weeks or in 8 females on Metrecal for 79-102 weeks.

Enovid added to the diet at 15 ppm (average intake, 30-40 µg/mouse/day) increased the mammary tumour incidence in castrated male (C3H x RIII)F_1 mice from 16 to 87% (10/61 and 20/23). The latent period for tumour development was decreased in both castrated males and ovariectomized females but the incidence in ovariectomized females was not significantly increased. In intact female RIII mice, Enovid had no effect on incidence or on latent period (Rudali, 1974).

Norethynodrel, when fed in the diet at 13.5 ppm (intake, 25-35 µg/mouse/day), altered neither the incidence nor the latent period of breast tumours in intact female RIII, C3H or (C3H x RIII)F_1 mice, nor in ovariectomized (C3H x RIII)F_1 females. In castrated males the breast tumour incidence was increased from 16 to 100%, and the latent period was reduced from an average of 82 to 37 weeks (Rudali, 1974).

Twenty female BALB/c mice were fed a liquid diet (Metrecal) containing an estimated dose of 10-12.5 µg of Enovid/mouse/day for an average period of 15 months. Of 16 mice which survived 10 months or more, 3 developed precancerous lesions and 2 developed squamous-cell carcinomas of the cervix and/or vagina. In addition, in a group of 40 mice treated with Enovid plus intravaginal inoculations of herpesvirus type 2, 31 mice survived 10 months or more; of these 1 developed a precancerous lesion and 6 developed squamous-cell carcinomas of the cervix and/or vagina. Among 15/20 control mice which survived 10 months or more, 1 precancerous lesion of the cervix was detected (Muñoz, 1973).

The Committee on Safety of Medicines (1972) coordinated a trial of norethynodrel alone or in combination with mestranol. The drugs were evaluated for carcinogenic activity by incorporation in the diet of one strain of mice for 80 weeks. The doses were identified only as low (2-5 times the human dose), medium (50-150 times) and high (200-400 times). The amounts were not specified. In groups of 120 CF-LP strain mice of each sex norethynodrel alone or in combination with mestranol (66:1 and 25:1) increased the incidence of pituitary tumours in males and females from a range of 2-8 in control groups to incidences of 30-47 in the treated groups. Most of the increased incidences were related to the medium and high doses. Small numbers of benign adrenal tumours were found. Malignant mammary tumours occurred in 5/40 female mice receiving the high dose of norethynodrel alone, compared with 4/240 controls.

Rat: The Committee on Safety of Medicines (1972) (see under "mouse" for details) concluded that norethynodrel alone increased the incidence of benign liver-cell tumours in groups of 120 male rats from 3 to 24%. This increase occurred mainly in animals administered the medium and high dose levels; malignant hepatomas occurred in 8% of the 120 males, mainly in animals receiving the medium and high doses. Norethynodrel with mestranol (66:1) induced a similar increase in incidence of benign liver-cell tumours (29%) in males, but the increase in malignant tumours (2% compared to 0% in the controls) is of doubtful significance. Female rats on the same treatments had much lower incidences of benign liver-cell tumours (<5%) and no malignant liver-cell tumours. Norethynodrel alone induced pituitary tumours in 43% of the 120 male rats (compared to 6% in controls) and norethynodrel plus mestranol at 25:1, but not at 66:1 (2%), also increased the incidence in males to 15%. Female rats ingesting norethynodrel alone had no incidence of pituitary tumours, but such tumours occurred in 20% of female rats fed norethynodrel plus mestranol (25:1), compared with 8% in controls. Both benign and malignant mammary tumours were induced by norethynodrel with or without mestranol in male rats (15-19% of rats had malignant mammary tumours, compared with 0% in controls), but in female rats the incidence of malignant tumours was increased only in the groups fed norethynodrel with mestranol (25:1) (20%, compared with 7% in controls). It was stated, but not tabulated, that these increases occurred almost entirely in the high dose group.

In a group of 21 female Wistar rats given gastric instillations of 3 mg Enovid 6 times/week for 50 weeks no breast tumours developed. The same treatment in a further group of 47 rats neither increased nor decreased the induction of tumours by 3-methylcholanthrene (Gruenstein et al., 1964). Administration of Enovid in sesame oil by gavage caused a small inhibition of the induction of breast tumours by 7,12-dimethylbenz(a)anthracene (DMBA) (Weisburger er al., 1968; Stern & Mickey, 1969). Daily administration of 0.25 mg Enovid by gavage in corn oil for 10 days prior to the administration of a single dose of 8 mg DMBA to intact female Sprague-Dawley rats increased the incidence of breast cancer to 81%, compared to 45% in the controls receiving DMBA only. Pretreatment for 10 days with 1 mg Enovid did not affect the subsequent tumour incidence (McCarthy, 1965).

Monkey: In a study still in progress at the time of reporting, an adenocarcinoma of the breast arose in 1/6 female rhesus monkeys after 18 months of daily feeding of 1 mg Enovid. There were widespread metastases (Kirschstein et al., 1972). {Assessment of this result is made difficult by the fact that the animals were 6-8 years old at the beginning of treatment and had borne at least one infant. However, the incidence of spontaneous breast cancer in monkeys of this colony was reported to be very low.}

(b) Subcutaneous and/or intramuscular injection

Rat: Repeated s.c. injections of 10 or 100 µg Enovid/day in corn oil into 2 groups of 25 female Sprague-Dawley rats for 40 days reduced the number of mammary tumours/rat produced by a single injection of 5 mg DMBA given on day 25 of treatment. The average number of tumours/rat was 10.9 in 37 controls given DMBA alone, compared with 7.6 and 3.9 in rats given 10 or 100 µg Enovid, respectively (Welsch & Meites, 1969).

Hamster: Twice-weekly s.c. injections of Enovid in sesame oil (34 mg/kg bw), reduced to 17 mg/kg bw at 94 weeks and to 8 mg/kg bw at 104 weeks, did not increase the incidence of any tumour type in 46 male hamsters. {However, the average age of the animals at the start of the experiment was 76 weeks, and 50% of the animals had died by 103 weeks.} (Sichuk et al., 1967).

(c) Subcutaneous implantation

Mouse: Lipschütz et al. (1966, 1967) reported 2 so-called granulosa-cell tumours of the ovaries among 24 female BALB/c mice implanted s.c. with pellets containing 40% norethynodrel and 60% cholesterol. The daily absorption was estimated to be 4-8 µg/day.

3.2 Other relevant biological data

See section, "General Remarks on the Sex Hormones", and pp. 38-40.

3.3 Observations in man

See section, "Oestrogens and Progestins in Relation to Human Cancer", p. 219.

4. Comments on Data Reported and Evaluation[1]

4.1 Animal data

Norethynodrel was tested alone or in combination with mestranol by the oral route in mice and rats. Alone, it was also tested by subcutaneous implantation in mice; and in combination with mestranol, by subcutaneous injection in rats. A subcutaneous injection study in hamsters and a feeding study in monkeys were of too limited duration to be considered for evaluation.

---

[1] This section should be read in conjunction with the section, "General Conclusions on Hormones", p. 235.

When given alone, norethynodrel increased the incidence of pituitary tumours in mice of both sexes and of mammary tumours in castrated males of one strain; it also increased the incidence of liver-cell, pituitary and mammary tumours in male rats.

In combination with mestranol, it increased the incidence of pituitary, vaginal and cervical tumours in female mice, of pituitary tumours in male mice, of mammary tumours in castrated male mice, of benign liver-cell tumours in male rats and of malignant mammary tumours in rats of both sexes.

4.2 Human data

No case reports or epidemiological studies on norethynodrel alone were available to the Working Group. Epidemiological studies on steroid hormones used in oestrogen-progestin contraceptive preparations have been summarized in the section, "Oestrogens and Progestins in Relation to Human Cancer", p. 223.

5. References

Blacow, N.W., ed. (1972) *Martindale. The Extra Pharmacopoeia*, 26th ed., London, The Pharmaceutical Press

Committee on Safety of Medicines (1972) *Carcinogenicity tests of oral contraceptives*, London, HMSO

Dunn, T.B. (1969) Cancer of the uterine cervix in mice fed a liquid diet containing an antifertility drug. *J. nat. Cancer Inst.*, 43, 671

Gruenstein, M., Shay, H. & Shimkin, M.B. (1964) Lack of effect of norethynodrel (Enovid) on methylcholanthrene-induced mammary carcinogenesis in female rats. *Cancer Res.*, 24, 1656-1658

Kastrup, E.K., ed. (1973) *Facts and Comparisons*, St. Louis, Missouri, Facts & Comparisons Inc.

Kirschstein, R.L., Rabson, A.S. & Rusten, G.W. (1972) Infiltrating duct carcinoma of the mammary gland of a rhesus monkey after administration of an oral contraceptive: a preliminary report. *J. nat. Cancer Inst.*, 48, 551-556

Lipschütz, A., Iglesias, R., Salinas, S. & Panasevich, V.I. (1966) Experimental conditions under which contraceptive steroids may become toxic. *Nature (Lond.)*, 212, 686-688

Lipschütz, A., Iglesias, R., Panasevich, V.I. & Salinas, S. (1967) Ovarian tumours and other ovarian changes induced in mice by two 19-nor-contraceptives. *Brit. J. Cancer*, 21, 153-159

McCarthy, J.D. (1965) Influence of two contraceptives on induction of mammary cancer in rats. *Amer. J. Surg.*, 110, 720-723

Muñoz, N. (1973) Effect of herpesvirus type 2 and hormonal imbalance on the uterine cervix of the mouse. *Cancer Res.*, 33, 1504-1508

Poel, W.E. (1966) Pituitary tumors in mice after prolonged feeding of synthetic progestins. *Science*, 154, 402-403

Rudali, G. (1974) Induction of tumors in mice with synthetic sex hormones. *Gann Monograph* (in press)

Sichuk, G., Fortner, J.G. & Der, B.K. (1967) Evaluation of the influence of norethynodrel with mestranol (Enovid) in middle-aged male Syrian (golden) hamsters, with particular reference to spontaneous tumours. *Acta Endocr.*, 55, 97-107

Stern, E. & Mickey, M.R. (1969) Effects of a cyclic steroid contraceptive regimen on mammary gland tumor induction in rats. *Brit. J. Cancer*, 23, 391-400

Weisburger, J.H., Weisburger, E.K., Griswold, D.P., Jr & Casey, A.E. (1968) Reduction of carcinogen-induced breast cancer in rats by an antifertility drug. Life Sci., 7, 259-266

Welsch, C.W. & Meites, J. (1969) Effects of a norethynodrel-mestranol combination (Enovid) on development and growth of carcinogen-induced mammary tumors in female rats. Cancer, 23, 601-607

NORGESTREL

1. Chemical and Physical Data

1.1 Synonyms and trade names*

Chem. Abstr. No.: 79-76-37

13-Ethyl-17α-ethynylgon-4-en-17β-ol-3-one; 13-ethyl-17α-ethynyl-17β-hydroxy-4-gonen-3-one; 13β-ethyl-17α-ethynyl-17-hydroxygon-4-en-3-one; 13β-ethyl-17α-ethynyl-17β-hydroxygon-4-en-3-one; (±)-13-ethyl-17α-ethynyl-17-hydroxygon-4-en-3-one; 13-ethyl-17-hydroxy-18,19-dinor-17α-pregn-4-en-20-yn-3-one; (±)-13-ethyl-17-hydroxy-18,19-dinor-17α-pregn-4-en-20-yn-3-one; 13-ethyl-17-hydroxy(17α)-18,19-dinorpregn-4-en-20-yn-3-one; 17-ethynyl-18-methyl-19-nortestosterone; 17β-hydroxy-18-methyl-19-nor-17α-pregn-4-en-20-yn-3-one; 18-methyl-17α-ethynyl-19-nortestosterone; d-norgestrel; d(-)-norgestrel; D-norgestrel

Duoluton; Eugynon; Eugynon 21; Eugynon 28; Eugynon ED; Evanor; Folinett; Follinyl; Neogentrol; Neogynon; Neogynon 21; Neogynon 28; Neogynon ED; Neovlar 21; Nordiol 28; Ovral; Ovran; Primovlar 21; Primovlar 28; Stediril; Stediril D; TSP-6;

1.2 Chemical formula and molecular weight

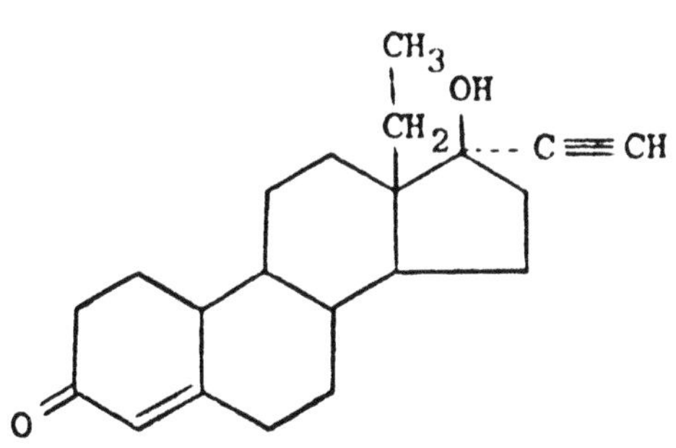

$C_{21}H_{28}O_2$
Mol. wt: 312.5

---

* Trade names include mixtures containing norgestrel

1.3 **Chemical and physical properties of the pure substance**

   (a) Description: White crystals

   (b) Melting-point: 206°C

   (c) Solubility: Practically insoluble in water; slightly soluble at 25°C in ethanol; soluble in acetone, chloroform and dioxane

1.4 **Technical products and impurities**

Norgestrel is available in the United States only in combination with ethinyloestradiol as tablets for use as oral contraceptives (Kastrup, 1973).

2. Production, Use, Occurrence and Analysis

2.1 **Production and use**[1]

A method for the synthesis of norgestrel was reported by Edgren et al. (1963); it is believed to be produced by total synthesis from non-steroid starting materials. In one method, 6-methoxy-1-tetralone is treated with vinylmagnesium bromide to form 6-methoxy-1-vinyl-1,2,3,4-tetrahydro-1-naphthol. This compound is condensed with 2-ethyl-1,3-cyclopentanedione to give 3-methoxy-8(14)-secooestra-1,3,5(10),9(11)-tetraen-13-ethyl-18-nor-14,17-dione, which is made to undergo a ring closure to give the steroid skeleton. The 17-keto group is reduced with sodium borohydride, and the 14(15)-double bond is reduced with hydrogen over palladium on carbon. A Birch reduction is then used to reduce the 8(9)-double bond and the 1- and 4- positions of the A ring. Oxidation of the alcohol is used to introduce a keto-group at the 17-position. Treatment with acetylene gives the 17-ethynyl carbinol, and hydrolysis of the 3-enol ether gives norgestrel. Whether this is the synthesis route used for commercial production is not known.

No data are available on the quantity of norgestrel produced by the only US manufacturer.

---

[1] Data from Chemical Information Services, Stanford Research Institute, USA

Norgestrel has been used in the US since 1968 as the progestin in progestin-oestrogen combination therapy oral contraceptive products (the oestrogen used in the US is ethinyloestradiol). Total US sales of norgestrel for use in oral contraceptives are estimated to be less than 200 kg annually.

In mid-1972, one source reported that the manufacturer of norgestrel was awaiting approval by the US Food and Drug Administration of a "mini-pill" said to contain noregestrel as the only active ingredient (Anon, 1972). The present status of this application is not known.

Data on production of norgestrel in the countries of Western Europe are not available, but production and sales are believed to be concentrated in a small number of companies. Total sales of norgestrel in hormone and contraceptive specialties in Western Europe in 1972 are estimated to have been less than 70 kg. Sales in France represented approximately 60% of the total, with lesser amounts sold in Italy, The Netherlands and the United Kingdom.

2.2 Occurrence

Norgestrel does not occur in nature.

2.3 Analysis

General methods of analysis are given in the section, "General Remarks on the Sex Hormones", p. 43.

3. Biological Data Relevant to the Evaluation of Carcinogenic Risk to Man

3.1 Carcinogenicity and related studies in animals

(a) Oral administration

Mouse: The Committee on Safety of Medicines (1972) coordinated a trial of norgestrel alone or in combination with ethinyloestradiol. The drugs were evaluated for carcinogenic activity by incorporation in the diet of one strain of mice for 80 weeks. The doses were identified only as low (2-5 times the human dose), medium (50-150 times) and high (200-400 times).

The amounts were not specified. Norgestrel administered alone or in combination with ethinyloestradiol (10:1) to groups of 120 male and 120 female CF-LP mice did not alter the incidence of tumours in any tissue compared with that in controls.

Rat: The Committee on Safety of Medicines (1972) (see under "mouse") considered the results of norgestrel administered alone or in combination with ethinyloestradiol (10:1) to groups of 120 male and 120 female Wistar rats. There was no alteration in the incidence of tumours in any tissue cmopared with that in 80 male and 80 female controls.

3.2 Other relevant biological data

See section, "General Remarks on the Sex Hormones", and pp. 38-40.

3.3 Observations in man

See section, "Oestrogens and Progestins in Relation to Human Cancer", p. 219.

4. Comments on Data Reported and Evaluation[1]

4.1 Animal data

Norgestrel was tested in one experiment only in mice and rats by the oral route. There was no increase in the incidence of tumours in either species compared with that in controls. Comparable results were obtained when norgestrel was administered in combination with ethinyloestradiol.

4.2 Human data

No case reports or epidemiological studies on norgestrel alone were available to the Working Group. Epidemiological studies on steroid hormones used in oestrogen-progestin contraceptive preparations have been summarized in the section, "Oestrogens and Progestins in Relation to Human Cancer", p. 223.

---

[1] This section should be read in conjunction with the section "General Conclusions on Hormones", p. 235.

5. References

Anon. (1972) The Wall Street Transcript, July 17, pp. 29,259-29,261

Committee on Safety of Medicines (1972) Carcinogenicity tests of oral contraceptives, London, HMSO

Edgren, R.A., Smith, H., Peterson, D.L. & Carter, D.L. (1963) The biological effects of a series of 13β-substituted gonanes related to norethisterone (17α-ethynyl-19-nortestosterone). Steroids, 2, 319-335

Kastrup, E.K., ed. (1973) Facts and Comparisons, St. Louis, Missouri, Facts & Comparisons Inc.

ANDROGENS

TESTOSTERONE

1. Chemical and Physical Data

1.1 Synonyms and trade names*

Chem. Abstr. No.: 58-22-0

Δ^4-Androsten-17β-ol-3-one; androst-4-en-17β-ol-3-one; Δ^4-androsten-17β-ol-3-one; 4-androsten-17β-ol-3-one; 17β-hydroxy-Δ^4-androsten-3-one; 17β-hydroxy androst-4-en-3-one; 17β-hydroxy-4-androsten-3-one; 17-hydroxy-(17β)-androst-4-en-3-one; trans-testosterone; testosterone hydrate; testostosterone

Ablacton; Androfort; Androlin; Andronaq; Andronoq; Androtest; Andrusol; Anertan; Aquaviron; Climanosid; Climaterine; Clivion; Combidurin; Cycladiene; Cycladiene M. Test.; Estandron; Estandron Prolong.; Foliteston; Foliteston Retard; Géno-cristaux Gremy; Gineserpina; Heptylate de Test.; Hormoduvadilan; Homosteron; Homosterone; Klimanosid R; Lutestex; Malestrone; Mertestate; Neo-Hombreol; Neotestis; Oreton; Oreton-F; Orquisteron; Perandren; Percutacrine Androgénique; Primodian D; Primodian Depot; Primotest; Primoteston; Sterandryl; Sustanon; Synandrol; Synandrol-F; Teslen; Testandrone; Test.-Folliculline; Testiculosterone; Testobase; Test.-Oestr. R; Testo Folicular; Testo Luteinica; Testoluton; Testosid; Testosteroid; Testosterona; Testoviron; Testoviron Schering; Testoviron Prog.; Testrone; Testryl; Trioestrine; Trioestrine R; Trioestrine Vitam.; Virormone; Virosterone

---

*Trade names include mixtures containing testosterone

1.2 Chemical formula and molecular weight

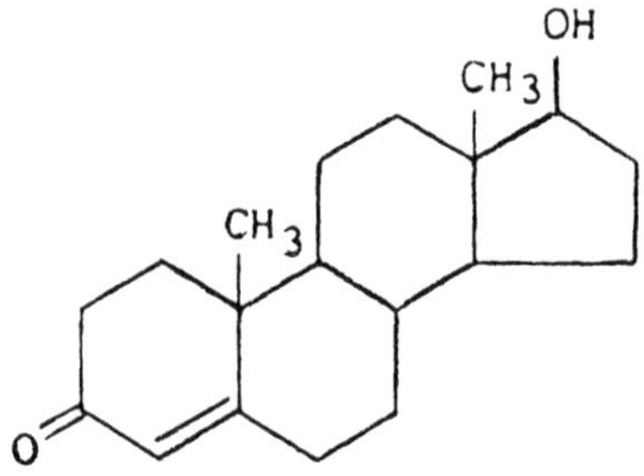

$C_{19}H_{28}O_2$

Mol. wt: 288.4

1.3 Chemical and physical properties of the pure substance

(a) Description: White needles (from dilute, aqueous acetone)

(b) Melting-point: 155°C

(c) Absorption spectrometry: λ_{max} 238 nm

(d) Optical rotation: $\{\alpha\}_D^{24}$ +109° (4% w/v in alcohol)

(e) Solubility: Very slightly soluble in water; soluble at 25°C in 95% ethanol (1 in 5), chloroform (1 in 2), ether (1 in 100); also soluble in acetone, dioxane and oils

1.4 Technical products and impurities

Testosterone is available in the United States as an aqueous injection and as pellets. It is also available as injections in combination with (1) Vitamin B1 and l-glutamic acid and (2) oestrone, oestrogenic substance or oestradiol-17β. Solutions of the cypionate (cyclopentylpropionate), oenanthate (heptanate) and propionate ester derivatives in vegetable oil are also available in several concentrations as injections, as are combinations of the cypionate with oestradiol cypionate and of the oenanthate with oestradiol valerate. The propionate is also available as tablets and as an injection in combination with oestradiol benzoate (Kastrup, 1973).

2. Production, Use, Occurrence and Analysis

2.1 Production and use[1]

Isolation of testosterone was first reported in 1935 by David et al. (Merck & Co.), and numerous methods of synthesis from other steroids (e.g., cholesterol) were subsequently reported. The single US manufacturer is believed to produce it from intermediates obtained by the degradation of diosgenin. In one method, degradation produces dehydroepiandrosterone, which is converted to testosterone by Oppenauer oxidation.

The US company which produces testosterone also produces the oenanthate and propionate esters. Another US company produces the cypionate ester. No data are available on the quantity of these chemicals produced in the US.

Testosterone (the most active of the natural androgens) and its ester derivatives are used in human medicine as androgenic, anabolic and anti-oestrogenic hormones for the treatment of a variety of conditions in both males and females. In males, they are used for the treatment of conditions due to androgen deficiency, delayed puberty, eunuchism, hypogonadism, impotence and oligospermia. In females, they are used for treatment of postpartum breast pain and engorgement and mammary cancer. They are used in both sexes as adjunct therapy for treatment of osteoporosis. Combinations of testosterone and its esters with oestrogens (e.g., oestradiol-17β, oestrone) are used for the treatment of menopausal symptoms, to control sodium retention, to inhibit lactation and prevent postpartum breast pain and engorgement and as adjunct therapy for treatment of postmenopausal and senile osteoporosis (Kastrup, 1973). Total US sales of testosterone and its ester derivatives for use in human medicine are estimated to be less than 500 kg annually.

Data on production of testosterone in the countries of Western Europe are not available, but it is known that one company in France manufactures

---

[1] Data from Chemical Information Services, Stanford Research Institute, USA

the chemical. Total sales of testosterone in hormone specialties in Western Europe in 1972 are estimated to have been less than 200 kg. Sales in France represented approximately 60% of the total, with lesser amounts sold in Spain and The Netherlands.

Until May 3, 1973, when the US Food and Drug Administration (FDA) banned their use, subcutaneous ear injections of a combination of testosterone and diethylstilboestrol were permitted in the US for the stimulation of growth and rate of finishing of beef cattle (US Environmental Protection Agency, 1973). Subcutaneous ear implants of a combination of testosterone propionate and oestradiol benzoate are still approved for use in the US to promote growth and feed efficiency in heifers (US Code of Federal Regulations, 1973). The quantity of testosterone propionate used in this way may have increased dramatically in recent months as a result of the FDA ban mentioned above.

Veterinary uses of testosterone include the treatment of cryptorchidism, impotence, mammary tumours in bitches, testicular deficiency and for the suppression of lactation (Merck & Co., 1968). No data are available on the quantity of testosterone and its ester derivatives consumed in the US for these purposes.

2.2 Occurrence

Testosterone is a widely occurring natural androgen (see section, "General Remarks on the Sex Hormones", p. 30, for further information).

2.3 Analysis

General methods of analysis are given in the section, "General Remarks on the Sex Hormones", p. 40.

3. Biological Data Relevant to the Evaluation of Carcinogenic Risk to Man

3.1 Carcinogenicity and related studies in animals

(a) Subcutaneous and/or intramuscular injection

Mouse: Schenken & Burns (1943) reported that s.c. injection of 0.25-1.25 mg/week of testosterone propionate in sesame oil for life or 25 weeks completely inhibited the spontaneous appearance of hepatomas in 24 male C3H mice. The incidence in 16 untreated, non-breeding males of this strain was 6%. Virgin females showed no significant incidence of hepatomas with or without testosterone injection.

Jones (1941) found a reduced incidence of mammary tumours (3/12) in virgin female C3H mice (with the MTV) injected s.c. with 1.0-1.5 mg of testosterone weekly in olive oil, after 20 months, compared with 18/38 in controls after 12 months. Gardner (1946) reported that testosterone propionate injected s.c., in doses ranging from 0.625 to 2.5 µg weekly, reduced the incidence of mammary cancers occurring in 88 male and 92 female C3H mice also given oestradiol benzoate in doses ranging from 3.3 to 33.3 µg weekly. A total of 17 mice developed mammary tumours, with an average latent period of 61 weeks, compared with 51/118 given the oestrogen alone, the average latent period being in this case 46 weeks.

Newborn mouse: Female BALB/cCrgl mice injected s.c. with 25 µg testosterone daily for the first 5 days after birth developed vaginal tumours in 7/9 animals at about 71 weeks of age (Kimura & Nandi, 1967). Thus, neonatal injections of androgen appear to act similarly to injections of oestradiol-17β (Takasugi et al., 1970). Neonatal exposure to testosterone is even more effective than that to oestradiol-17β in increasing mammary tumour incidence in MTV-bearing female BALB/cf C3H mice: 88% of androgen-treated mice showed mammary tumours at a mean age of 8.5 months (Bern et al., 1973).

Rat: Horning (1958) injected 20 female albino rats s.c. from the age of 3 days with 0.5 mg testosterone propionate weekly, increasing the doses to 2.5 mg at 6 months of age. Nine rats died during the first 6 months. Of 10 rats which survived 16 months or more of continuous treatment 3 had thecal-cell ovarian tumours. The pituitaries were not enlarged, but there was marked epithelial hyperplasia in the uteri of 5/10 rats. Neither ovarian nor uterine tumours occurred in untreated rats of that colony.

Hamster: Kirkman (1957) summarized the characteristics of three types of tumours (numbers not given) induced in Syrian hamsters by a combined treatment with s.c. injection or s.c. implantation of oestrogen plus testosterone. One of three tumour types arose from the uterine endometrium, the second from the vas deferens-epididymis, and the third type was a basal cell epithelioma arising in the flank. All these tumours retained a dependence for growth on a combination of oestrogen with testosterone. The first two tumour types do not occur in untreated hamsters.

(b) Subcutaneous implantation

Mouse: The incidence of leukaemia in 36 ovariectomized female Rockefeller Institute mice implanted with 3 mg pellets of testosterone propionate and observed up to 55 weeks was 58%, compared with 88% in 26 untreated, intact females and 90% in 31 untreated, ovariectomized females (Murphy, 1944).

van Nie et al. (1961) found cervical-uterine tumours in 26/42 (C57BL x dba)F_1 mice implanted with 1-2 mg pellets of testosterone propionate twice weekly for lifespan. The tumours were infiltrating and metastasized to the lungs in 10 mice.

Hamster: Kirkman (1957) summarized the characteristics of three types of tumours (numbers not given) induced in Syrian hamsters by a combined treatment with s.c. injection or s.c. implantation of oestrogen plus testosterone (see under "Subcutaneous and/or intramuscular injection").

Rivière et al. (1961) reported the induction by s.c. implantation (twice in 11 months) of pellets containing 100 mg testosterone propionate and 25 mg diethylstilboestrol dipropionate of leiomyomas and leiomyosarcomas along the uterine horns in 18/20 females and of similar tumours in the epididymis of 17/20 males. Similar tumours were described by Kirkman & Algard (1965).

3.2 Other relevant biological data

See section, "General Remarks on the Sex Hormones", and pp. 38-40.

3.3 Observations in man

Johnson et al. (1972) described 4 patients with aplastic anaemia who developed hepatocellular carcinoma after long-term therapy with androgenic-anabolic steroids (testosterone derivatives). These findings are difficult to interpret because liver conditions such as hemosiderosis and hepatitis, which may be associated with hepatocellular carcinoma, have frequently been described in patients with aplastic anaemia.

4. Comments on Data Reported and Evaluation[1]

4.1 Animal data

Testosterone was tested by subcutaneous injection and/or implantation in mice, rats and hamsters.

Testosterone implanted subcutaneously induced cervical-uterine tumours in mice, which metastasized in some cases. The only study in rats was considered inadequate in numbers of animals.

The incidences of leukaemia and of liver-cell and breast tumours in untreated mice of some strains were decreased by testosterone treatment, but the incidence of mammary tumours was increased by neonatal treatment of females of a mammary-tumour-virus-bearing strain.

Three distinctive types of neoplasm were induced in hamsters by a combination of oestrogen and testosterone: a tumour of the uterine endometrium, a tumour of the vas deferens-epididymis and a basal-cell epithelioma of the flank. They remained dependent on oestrogen and testosterone for continued growth.

4.2 Human data

No adequate epidemiological data on testosterone alone were available to the Working Group.

---

[1] This section should be read in conjunction with the section, "General Conclusions on Hormones", p. 235.

5. References

Bern, H.A., Mori, T. & Young, P.N. (1973) Preliminary report on the effects of perinatal exposure to hormones on the mammary gland of female BALB/cf.C3H mice. In: Proceedings of the 8th Meeting on Mammary Cancer in Experimental Animals and Man, Airlie House, Virginia, p. 12

Gardner, W.U. (1946) The incidence of mammary tumors and the structure of mammary glands of estrogen-plus-testosterone-treated mice. Cancer Res., 6, 493

Horning, E.S. (1958) Carcinogenic action of androgens. Brit. J. Cancer, 12, 414-418

Jones, E.E. (1941) The effect of testosterone propionate on mammary tumors in mice of the C3H strain. Cancer Res., 1, 787-789

Johnson, F.L., Feagler, J.R., Lerner, K.G., Majerus, P.W., Siegel, M., Hartman, J.R. & Thomas, E.D. (1972) Association of androgenic-anabolic steroid therapy with development of hepatocellular carcinoma. Lancet, ii, 1273-1276

Kastrup, E.K., ed. (1973) Facts and Comparisons, St. Louis, Missouri, Facts & Comparisons Inc.

Kimura, T. & Nandi, S. (1967) Nature of induced persistent vaginal cornification in mice. IV. Changes in the vaginal epithelium of old mice treated neonatally with estradiol or testosterone. J. nat. Cancer Inst., 39, 75-93

Kirkman, H. (1957) Steroid tumorigenesis. Cancer, 10, 757-764

Kirkman, H. & Algard, F.T. (1965) Characteristics of an androgen/estrogen-induced dependent leiomyosarcoma of the ductus deferens of the Syrian hamster. Cancer Res., 25, 141-143

Merck & Co. (1968) The Merck Index, 8th ed., Rahway, N.J., pp. 1020-1021

Murphy, J.B. (1944) The effect of castration, theelin and testosterone on the incidence of leukemia in a Rockefeller Institute strain of mice. Cancer Res., 4, 622-624

van Nie, R., Benedetti, E.L. & Mühlbock, O. (1961) A carcinogenic action of testosterone, provoking uterine tumours in mice. Nature (Lond.), 192, 1303

Rivière, M.R., Chouroulinkov, I. & Guérin, M. (1961) Actions hormonales expérimentales de longue durée chez le hamster du point de vue de leur effet cancérigène. II. Etude de la testostérone associée à un oestrogène. Bull. Cancer, 48, 499-524

Schenken, J.R. & Burns, E.L. (1943) Spontaneous primary hepatomas in mice of strain C3H. III. The effect of estrogens and testosterone propionate on their incidence. Cancer Res., 3, 693-696

Takasugi, N., Kimura, J. & Mori, J. (1970) Irreversible changes in mouse vaginal epithelium induced by early post-natal treatment with steroid hormones. In: Kazda, S. & Denenberg, V.H., eds, The Post-natal Development of Phenotype, Prague, Academia, pp. 229-251

US Code of Federal Regulations (1973) Washington DC, US Government Printing Office, 21 CFR 135b.5

US Environmental Protection Agency (1973) Tolerances for residues for new animal drugs in food. Federal Register, 38, No. 85, Washington DC, US Government Printing Office, pp. 10,926-10,927

OESTROGENS AND PROGESTINS IN RELATION TO HUMAN CANCER

The possible role of oestrogens and progestins in relation to human cancer has been discussed among others by Allen (1969), Dodds (1961) and Hertz (1968).

A considerable variety of observations have suggested that there is a relationship between endogenously produced female sex hormones and neoplasms of the breast or of the reproductive system. The following discussion, however, will be limited to administered exogenous hormones.

Some of the data concerned with specific agents are mentioned and discussed in the monographs. The following is a discussion of observations in man which cannot be attributed to the effect of a single substance.

The examination of trends in the incidence of cancer of the female reproductive organs and breast will not be discussed here, since these malignancies have been shown to bear an epidemiological relationship to various aspects of sexual and reproductive behaviour, which are undergoing changes in many parts of the world. Furthermore, the availability and use of newer diagnostic methods and screening procedures has increased markedly. These factors make it impossible to ascribe to the use of oestrogens or oral contraceptives any changes in incidence that have been observed to date.

Oestrogens used in treatment

Case reports of the occurrence of cancer of the breast or reproductive organs in women who have received oestrogen treatment are of little or no significance, because these diseases are common, and oestrogen treatment has been widespread for many years. However, breast cancer has been reported in two male transvestites who took oestrogens in large doses to produce gynaecomastia (Symmers, 1968). The disease in young men and the treatment are both so rare that it is difficult to believe that the events were not causally related. The question of the possible relationship between diethylstilboestrol therapy for carcinoma of the prostate and cancer of the male breast is discussed on page 68.

A number of uncontrolled follow-up studies of groups of women receiving long-term oestrogen therapy for such conditions as the menopausal syndrome, senile vaginitis and osteoporosis have been reported. The main features of these studies are summarized in Table VII. All are deficient in several respects. For example, no attention has been given to the influence of confounding factors (e.g., socio-economic status and age at first pregnancy) which are now known to be important in the epidemiology of cancer of the breast and cervix. Again, allowance has not been made for the reduced incidence of cancer which might be expected early during the follow-up period, resulting from the careful examinations made prior to the commencement of therapy. Furthermore, in none of the studies are any details given regarding the method and thoroughness of follow-up, and in most of them the closure date is not specified. In some of the papers no expected frequencies of cancer are provided for comparative purposes. In others, where expected numbers are provided, their derivation is obscure. Wilson (1962), for example, states that 18 cancers of the breast and reproductive system were expected in his study which covered only 2387 person-years of exposure among women who were, on average, 51 years old at entry to the study. Application of the data on cancer incidence recorded by the Connecticut Registry to Wilson's data would suggest that the true figure is likely to be nearer 7. Despite all the reservations, however, it cannot be denied that the incidence of cancer of the breast and of the reproductive system in the studies detailed in Table VII appears to be low; certainly they do not provide any evidence of a carcinogenic risk.

Wynder et al. (1960) conducted a case-control study on 632 female patients with breast cancer and on a like number of controls. They found no significant difference in the use of oestrogens between the two groups. The Boston Collaborative Drug Surveillance Program (1974) has also reported a case-control study relating to female patients aged 45-69 years of whom 51 had breast cancer, 52 had benign tumours of the breast and 774 were controls. Again, no association was found between oestrogen use and the breast lesions, either benign or malignant.

There is, however, evidence that the use of diethylstilboestrol for the management of gonadal dysgenesis in young women may predispose to the

TABLE VII

INCIDENCE OF CANCER OF THE BREAST AND REPRODUCTIVE SYSTEM IN RELATION TO LONG-TERM OESTROGEN ADMINISTRATION

Authors	Number of patients	Ages of patients	Number of hysterectomized patients at entry	Substances administered & duration of treatment	Duration of follow-up	Number & type of cancers observed (breast & reproductive system only)
Geist & Salmon (1941)	206	25-80	Not stated	Oestradiol compounds. Duration of therapy, 0.5-5.5 years	0.5-5.5 years	None
Wallach & Henneman (1959)	292	15-83 (mean, 51)	94 (total or partial hysterectomy	Oestradiol, diethylstilboestrol, conjugated equine-oestrogens 67 also received a progestational agent. Mean duration of therapy, 5.1 years	Up to 25 years	Endometrium - 4 Ovary - 2 Carcinoma-in situ of cervix - 1
Mustacchi & Gordon (1958)	120	15-84 (mean, 50)	Not stated	Conjugated equine-oestrogens, ethinyl-oestradiol, diethylstilboestrol, methallenoestril. Mean duration of therapy, 5 years	Mean, 5 years	None

TABLE VII (cont'd)

Authors	Number of patients	Ages of patients	Number of hysterectomized patients at entry	Substances administered & duration of treatment	Duration of follow-up	Number & type of cancers observed (breast & reproductive system only)
Wilson (1962)	304	40-73 (mean, 51)	86	Mostly conjugated equine-oestrogens. 83 also received a progestational agent. Mean duration of therapy, 7.8 years (1-27 years)	1-27 years (mean, 7.8 years)	None
Schleyer-Saunders (1966)	300	30-70	Not stated	Implants containing oestradiol, testosterone and deoxycortisone. Duration of therapy, "several years"	Up to 25 years	Breast - 3 Cervix - 2 Endometrium - 1 Ovary - 1
Leis (1966)	158	36-54 (mean, 46)	29	Conjugated equine-oestrogens. All also received progestational agents. Duration of therapy, 10-14 years	10-14 years	None
Burch & Byrd (1971)	511	27-72 (mean, 54)	511	Almost all received conjugated equine-oestrogens. Duration of therapy, "a long period of time"	9 years or more	Breast - 9

development of carcinoma of the endometrium (see page 68). Furthermore, there is indisputable evidence that the administration of diethylstilboestrol to women during pregnancy is associated with a risk of vaginal or cervical adenocarcinoma in their exposed female offspring (see page 66).

In a large, randomized trial of several drugs for the prevention of further attacks in men who had had a myocardial infarction (Coronary Drug Project Research Group, 1973), a suggestion of an increased incidence of cancer, especially of lung cancer, was seen among the men who received conjugated equine-oestrogens in dosages of 2.5 mg per day, as compared with those receiving placebos. The duration of exposure of the men who developed cancer is not stated in the report; it may be noted, however, that at the closure date for the analysis, the mean duration of exposure of all men in the oestrogen-treated group was 56 months.

Progestins used in treatment

No data were available to the Working Group.

Oestrogens and progestins used in oral contraceptives

CERVIX

A distinctive atypical polypoid endocervical hyperplasia of the cervix was described by Taylor et al. (1967) in 13 patients taking oral contraceptives for periods of up to 4 years. Apparently similar lesions were reported by Candy & Abell (1968) in 11 patients taking the same drugs. The histological descriptions and illustrations are suggestive of adenocarcinoma, and this was the initial diagnosis in some of the cases. Both reports emphasized that in the authors' opinion the lesions were benign and should be so treated. In another study, two distinct types of cervical epithelial hyperplasia, described as "epidermidalization" or microglandular hyperplasia, were described in detail by Kyriakos et al. (1968). Twenty-two of the 30 patients presenting such lesions were taking oral contraceptives. The authors were of the opinion that the lesions were induced by the preparations and were non-malignant, but that they could be confused with carcinoma.

A large number of other studies have been concerned with the effect of oral contraceptives on the cervical epithelium (Pincus & Garcia, 1965;

Attwood, 1966; Ayre et al., 1966; Maqueo et al., 1966; Wied et al., 1966; Liu et al., 1967; Gall et al., 1969; Melamed et al., 1969; Chai et al., 1970; Kline et al., 1970; Boyce et al., 1972; Thomas, 1972; Worth & Boyes, 1972; Fuertes-de la Haba et al., 1973). The findings have been inconsistent. Four of these papers, which appear to be the most adequate, have been selected for detailed consideration.

Melamed et al. (1969), in New York, compared the prevalence of carcinoma-in situ in 27,508 women choosing and using oral contraception and in 6809 choosing and using the diaphragm, attending 11 centres run by Planned Parenthood. The prevalence rate in the former group was twice as high as that in the latter group. It may be noted that this study was not prospective in character.

These findings are extremely difficult to interpret; however, it would appear that either (1) the oral contraceptives caused the development of carcinoma-in situ, (2) the use of a diaphragm protected against it, or (3) the women who chose to use oral contraceptives were more likely, for other reasons, to develop the lesion. In favour of the second possibility is evidence from retrospective studies (Rotkin & King, 1962; Boyd & Doll, 1964) that diaphragms may protect against carcinoma of the cervix. The third possibility is difficult to exclude. Melamed and his colleagues did their best to do so by dividing the women into groups according to their age, ethnic origins, age at first pregnancy, number of children and family income and by matching patients in the two contraceptive groups according to these characteristics. The results showed that the proportion of positive cases in the oral contraceptive group in 2351 matched pairs was significantly greater than in the diaphragm group. Since, however, matching was achieved only by considering broad categories, while the two contraceptive groups were extremely heterogenous with respect to the factors considered in the matching (Dubrow et al., 1969), this finding is much less conclusive than it might appear to be. It may also be relevant that in a study in California reported by Stern et al. (1970), women choosing oral contraceptives were found significantly more often to have cervical dysplasia before starting medication than those choosing other methods (8% versus 5%), and that this difference could not be attributed to religion, ethnic group, age, age at first intercourse, age at first pregnancy, number of children or family income.

Worth & Boyes (1972) reported a case-control study of carcinoma-<u>in situ</u> of the cervix, the cases being derived from a screening programme which covered about 80% of the adult female population of British Columbia. The study was limited to women in the third decade of life. Of 445 women with carcinoma-<u>in situ</u>, information was obtained for only 310. For each case, the controls were intended to be the next three age-matched women with negative smears seen in the practice of the physician responsible for the care of the case. In the event, information was obtained for only 682 controls. The data about contraceptive use, social history, etc. for both cases and controls were obtained by means of a questionnaire sent to the individual physicians. There were no significant differences in the frequency or duration of oral contraceptive use between the cases and controls. The two groups, however, differed greatly with respect to marital status and history of previous pregnancy, and no adjustment was made for these differences. It may also be noted that about 90% of the women included in the analysis, both cases and controls, were stated to have used oral contraceptives at some time.

Boyce et al. (1972) interviewed 196 consecutive patients with carcinoma of the cervix (151 <u>in situ</u>, 43 invasive and 2 unstaged) seen at the Downstate Medical Center in New York. Three-quarters of the patients were black. An equal number of controls with recent normal cervical smears was similarly interviewed. These controls were matched with the cases for age, ethnic background, age at first coitus, age at first pregnancy and socio-economic status. The source and method of selection of the controls, however, is inadequately described. No significant difference in the frequency or duration of oral contraceptive use was found between the cases and controls.

Thomas (1972) attempted to trace all white women aged 15-50 years in Washington County, Maryland having a cytological smear suggestive of neoplasia during the interval 1965-69 by searching the records of the Washington County General Hospital. He identified 378 such women and succeeded in interviewing 324. Of these, 104 had carcinoma-in situ, 105 had dysplasia, 25 had chronic inflammatory changes and 90 had no biopsy. For control purposes, he selected 360 women representing a 1 in 30 probability sample of the 15-50-year-old, white, female population of the county who had at least one smear on record at the hospital between 1965 and 1969. He succeeded in interviewing 302 of these women. There were no significant differences in the frequency or duration of oral contraceptive use between any of the subgroups of cases and the controls; however, 8 variables were identified which did differ significantly between the groups. Accordingly, Thomas computed relative risk estimates for the oral contraceptive data by a multiple regression technique which took into consideration these 8 variables and a further 5 which were thought possibly to be of importance. None of the relative risk estimates obtained in this way differed significantly from unity. Indeed the relative risk for carcinoma-in situ was 0.6, suggesting, if anything, a negative association between oral contraceptive use and this condition.

Mention must also be made of the study reported from Puerto Rico by Fuertes-de la Haba et al. (1973) which started in 1961 and is stated to be a double-blind trial measuring progression and regression of cervical cytological abnormalities among 4846 users of an oral contraceptive containing norethynodrel and mestranol and 4788 non-users of the preparations. Unfortunately, this study is extremely hard to interpret. First, it is difficult to see how the prescription of oral contraceptives could have been double-blind. Secondly, no information is provided about the subsequent adherence of the women to the contraceptive group to which they were originally allocated. Thirdly, no details about the adequacy of follow-up are given. Finally, the analysis groups together all women whose smear results changed from one diagnostic category to another, irrespective of the time at which the changes were observed and irrespective of whether these changes were, for example, from normal to atypia or from dysplasia to carcinoma-in situ. With these reservations, it may be noted that the study indicated no significant differences in the pattern of progression or regression between the oral and the non-oral groups.

In conclusion, there seems to be no convincing evidence at the present time that the use of oral contraceptives is related either positively or negatively to the risk of carcinoma-in situ of the cervix. However, the numbers of subjects in the more reliable studies are insufficient to detect a small change in risk. Furthermore, information on invasive carcinoma of the cervix is almost entirely lacking. It should also be noted that the duration of exposure to the preparation by most of the women included in the studies previously discussed is relatively short, and that oral contraceptives have been in widespread use for little more than a decade.

BREAST

The histopathological features of breast lesions excised from women using oral contraceptives have been described in several studies. Fechner (1970a,b,c) examined 54 fibroadenomas, 25 chronic fibrocystic disease specimens and 5 breast cancers obtained from women using the preparations. For control purposes, he selected corresponding pathological material from women without such exposure. In the case of the benign lesions, the histopathological assessment was made without knowlege as to which specimens were obtained from women using oral contraceptives. He found no distinctive features which he could relate to the use of the steroids.

Vessey et al. (1972) studied the pathological features of 255 benign lesions of the breast and of 90 breast cancers excised from women aged 16-39 years. The review was again conducted without knowledge of the patients' contraceptive habits. Their findings were in line with those of Fechner: it was impossible to distinguish lesions, benign or malignant, excised from the breasts of women using oral contraceptives from those excised from the breasts of women not doing so.

On the other hand, Goldenberg et al. (1968) and Brown (1970) reported on 4 patients and 1 patient, respectively, who were using oral contraceptives and who were treated for fibroadenomas showing a bizarre type of epithelial proliferation which these authors believed to be related to the use of the preparations. Wiegenstein et al. (1971) also reported that 11 of a series of 12 patients with multiple breast fibroadenomas, a rare phenomenon in their experience, had histories of one month to 5 years of oral contraceptive use.

A number of case-control epidemiological studies of the possible relationship between breast neoplasia and use of oral contraceptives or oestrogens have been reported. Arthes et al. (1971) in the United States made a report concerning three such studies. In the first of these there were 134 cases of breast cancer identified from a county cancer register, the majority of whom were diagnosed prior to 1963. There were two age-matched control groups: 121 neighbourhood controls and 139 women constituting a probability sample of the county population. In the second investigation, there were 30 cases of breast cancer under the age of 35 and 30 matched controls. The third investigation included 119 newly-diagnosed cases of breast cancer aged 15-75 years and an equal number of controls matched on age, race, marital status and partially on economic status. The controls were admitted for elective surgery to the same hospital as were the cases. In none of these 3 studies were any significant differences found between cases and controls in the frequency or duration of use of either oral contraceptives or of oestrogens.

The same group of workers (Sartwell et al., 1973) reported on the use of these drugs by 416 patients aged 15-75 having benign breast lesions, and by an equal number of controls. These data were acquired in the course of the third investigation described in the previous paragraph, in which the patients with breast lesions were interviewed preoperatively, before the benign or malignant character of their disease was known. The 416 controls were matched to the cases for the same factors as mentioned above. No major differences in the prior use of oral contraceptives or oestrogens between cases and controls were found.

Vessey et al. (1972), in the United Kingdom, interviewed 345 women aged 16-39 years with a lump in the breast, of whom 90 had cancer and 255 had benign lesions, together with 347 controls matched for age, marital status, hospital attended and parity. No significant differences were found in the frequency and duration of use of oral contraceptives between the patients with breast cancer and the controls. However, significantly fewer of the patients with fibroadenoma or chronic cystic disease gave a history of the use of the preparation than did the corresponding controls. This apparent protective effect was largely confined to women who were current users of oral contraceptives, with a total period of exposure exceeding two years. It was estimated that such women had only about 25% as great a risk of being admitted to hospital for a breast biopsy as women who had never used oral contraceptives at all.

The Boston Collaborative Drug Surveillance Program (1973) reported on 23 women with breast cancer, 98 with benign lesions of the breast and 842 control subjects. All these women were aged 20-44 years and were asked if they had used oral contraceptives during the previous 3 months. No matching was employed, but the comparisons were age adjusted. The proportion of women using oral contraceptives did not differ significantly between the breast cancer group and the control group. However, a significant negative association between the use of the preparations and benign breast lesions was found, and this was most pronounced in the women with fibroadenoma.

It may be concluded that at the present time there is no evidence to suggest that either oral contraceptives or oestrogen therapy have a role in the aetiology of breast cancer in the female. However, it should be strongly emphasized first that the studies reported to date include far too few patients to permit the detection of even a moderate change in risk and secondly that the time elapsed since the use of oral contraceptives became widespread may be insufficient to reveal such a change should it exist.

With regard to benign lesions of the breast, there is some reason to believe that oral contraceptives may have a protective effect.

LIVER

Baum et al. (1973) reported 7 cases of histologically benign hepatoma in the Michigan (US) area, and Contostavlos (1973) reported one more similar case from Pennsylvania (US); all 8 were in women aged 22-39 who had been using an oral contraceptive for a duration varying from 6 months to 7 years. All Baum's cases were detected or confirmed after clinical manifestations leading to surgery.

Benign hepatoma is a rare tumour; it is unlikely that the series of 7 cases described by Baum would occur by chance in the course of 5 years in the same area, and this suggests involvement of a new environmental factor, which may be the use of oral contraceptives.

5. References

Allen, W. (1969) Possible hazards in estrogen administration. Cancer, 24, 1137-1139

Arthes, F.G., Sartwell, P.E. & Lewison, E.F. (1971) The pill, estrogens and the breast. Epidemiologic aspects. Cancer, 28, 1391-1394

Attwood, M.E. (1966) Cytology and the contraceptive pill. J. Obstet. Gynaec. Brit. Cwlth, 73, 662-665

Ayre, J.E., Hillemanns, H.G., Le Guerrier, J. & Arsenault, J. (1966) Influence of norethynodrel and mestranol upon cervical dysplasia and carcinoma in situ. Obstet. Gynec., 28, 90-98

Baum, J.K., Holtz, F., Bookstein, J.J. & Klein, E.W. (1973) Possible association between benign hepatomas and oral contraceptives. Lancet, ii, 926-929

Boston Collaborative Drug Surveillance Program (1973) Oral contraceptives and venous thromboembolic disease, surgically confirmed gallbladder disease and breast tumours. Lancet, i, 1399-1404

Boston Collaborative Drug Surveillance Program (1974) Surgically confirmed gallbladder disease, venous thromboembolism and breast tumours in relation to postmenopausal estrogen therapy. New Engl. J. Med., 290, 15-18

Boyce, J.G., Lu, T., Nelson, J.H., Jr & Joyce, D. (1972) Cervical carcinoma and oral contraception. Obstet. Gynec., 40, 139-146

Boyd, J.T. & Doll, R. (1964) A study of the aetiology of carcinoma of the cervix uteri. Brit. J. Cancer, 18, 419-434

Brown, J.M. (1970) Histological modification of fibroadenoma of the breast associated with oral hormonal contraceptives. Med. J. Austr., i, 276-277

Burch, J.C. & Byrd, B.F., Jr (1971) Effects of long-term administration of estrogens on the occurrence of mammary cancer in women. Ann. Surg., 174, 414-418

Candy, M. & Abell, M.R. (1968) Progestogen-induced adenomatous hyperplasia of the uterine cervix. J. Amer. med. Ass., 203, 85-88

Chai, M.S., Johnson, W.D. & Tricomi, V. (1970) Five years' experience with contraceptive pills; cervical epithelial changes. N.Y. State J. Med., 70, 2663-2666

Contostavlos, D.L. (1973) Benign hepatomas and oral contraceptives. Lancet, ii, 1200

Coronary Drug Project Research Group (1973) The coronary drug project findings leading to discontinuation of the 2.5 mg/day estrogen group. J. Amer. med. Ass., 226, 652-657

Dodds, E.C. (1961) Rime and reason in endocrinology. In: Proceedings of the Society for Endocrinology, Eighty-fourth (ordinary) Meeting. J. Endocrinol., 23, i-xi

Dubrow, H., Melamed, M.R., Flehinger, B.J., Kelisky, R.P. & Koss, L.G. (1969) A study of factors affecting choice of contraceptives. Obstet. Gynec. Surv., 24, 1012-1022

Fechner, R.E. (1970a) Fibroadenomas in patients receiving oral contraceptives: a clinical and pathological study. Amer. J. clin. Path., 53, 857-864

Fechner, R.E. (1970b) Fibrocystic disease in women receiving oral contraceptive hormones. Cancer, 25, 1332-1339

Fechner, R.E. (1970c) Breast cancer during oral contraceptive therapy. Cancer, 26, 1204-1211

Fuertes-de la Haba, A., Pelegrina, I. Bangdiwala, I.S. & Hernández-Cibes, J.J. (1973) Changing patterns in cervical cytology among oral and non-oral contraceptive users. J. Reprod. Med., 10, 3-10

Gall, S.A., Bourgeois, C.H. & Maguire, R. (1969) The morphologic effects of oral contraceptive agents on the cervix. J. Amer. med. Ass., 207, 2243-2247

Geist, S.H. & Salmon, U.J. (1941) Are estrogens carcinogenic in the human female? The effect of long-continued estrogen administration upon the uterine and vaginal mucosa of the human female. Amer. J. Obstet. Gynec., 42, 29-36

Goldenberg, V.E., Wiegenstein, L. & Mottet, N.K. (1968) Florid breast fibroadenomas in patients taking hormonal oral contraceptives. Amer. J. clin. Path., 49, 52-59

Hertz, R. (1968) Experimental and clinical aspects of the carcinogenic potential of steroid contraceptives. Int. J. Fert., 13, 273-286

Kline, T.S., Holland, M. & Wemple, D. (1970) Atypical cytology with contraceptive hormone medication. Amer. J. clin. Path., 53, 215-222

Kyriakos, M., Kempson, R.L. & Konikov, N.F. (1968) A clinical and pathologic study of endocervical lesions associated with oral contraceptives. Cancer, 22, 99-110

Leis, H.P., Jr (1966) Endocrine prophylaxis of breast cancer with cyclic estrogen and progesterone. Int. Surg., 45, 496-503

Liu, W., Koebel, L., Shipp, J. & Prisby, H. (1967) Cytologic changes following the use of oral contraceptives. Obstet. Gynec., 30, 228-232

Maqueo, M., Azuela, J.C., Calderon, J.J. & Goldzieher, J.W. (1966) Morphology of the cervix in women treated with synthetic progestins. Amer. J. Obstet. Gynec., 96, 994-998

Melamed, M.R., Koss, L.G., Flehinger, B.J., Kelisky, R.P. & Dubrow, H. (1969) Prevalence rates of uterine cervical carcinoma in situ for women using the diaphragm or contraceptive oral steroids. Brit. med. J., iii, 195-200

Mustacchi, P. & Gordon, G.S. (1958) Frequency of cancer in estrogen-treated osteoporotic women. In: Segaloff, A., ed., Breast Cancer, the Second Biennial Louisiana Cancer Conference, New Orleans, St. Louis, C.V. Mosby & Co., pp. 163-169

Pincus, G. & Garcia, C.R. (1965) Studies on vaginal, cervical and uterine histology. Metabolism, 14, 344-347

Rotkin, I.D. & King, R.W. (1962) Environmental variables related to cervical cancer. Amer. J. Obstet. Gynec., 83, 720-728

Sartwell, P.E., Arthes, E.G. & Tonascia, J.A. (1973) Epidemiology of benign breast lesions: lack of association with oral contraceptive use. New Engl. J. Med., 288, 551-554

Schleyer-Saunders, E. (1966) The climacteric. A geriatric and social problem. In: Proceedings of the 7th International Congress of Gerontology, Vienna, 1966, Vienna, Wiener Medizinische Akademie, pp. 125-135

Stern, E., Clark, V.A. & Coffelt, C.F. (1970) Contraceptives and dysplasia: higher rate for pill choosers. Science, 169, 497-498

Symmers, W.St.C. (1968) Carcinoma of breast in trans-sexual individuals after surgical and hormonal interference with the primary and secondary sex characteristics. Brit. med. J., ii, 83-85

Taylor, H.B., Irey, N.S. & Norris, H.J. (1967) Atypical endocervical hyperplasia in women taking oral contraceptives. J. Amer. med. Ass., 202, 185-187

Thomas, D.B. (1972) Relationship of oral contraceptives to cervical carcinogenesis. Obstet. Gynec., 40, 508-518

Vessey, M.P., Doll, R. & Sutton, P.M. (1972) Oral contraceptives and breast neoplasia: a retrospective study. Brit. med. J., iii, 719-724

Wallach, S. & Henneman, P.H. (1959) Prolonged estrogen therapy in post-menopausal women. J. Amer. med. Ass., 171, 1637-1642

Wied, G.L., Davis, M.E., Frank, R., Segal, P.B., Meier, P. & Rosenthal, E. (1966) Statistical evaluation of the effect of hormonal contraceptives on the cytologic smear pattern. Obstet. Gynec., 27, 327-334

Wiegenstein, L., Tank, R. & Gould, V.E. (1971) Multiple breast fibroadenomas in women on hormonal contraceptives. New Engl. J. Med., 284, 676

Wilson, R.A. (1962) The roles of estrogen and progesterone in breast and genital cancer. J. Amer. med. Ass., 182, 327-331

Worth, A.J. & Boyes, D.A. (1972) A case-control study into the possible effects of birth control pills on pre-clinical carcinoma of the cervix. J. Obstet. Gynaec. Brit. Cwlth, 79, 673-679

Wynder, E.L., Bross, I.J. & Hirayama, T. (1960) A study of the epidemiology of cancer of the breast. Cancer, 13, 559-601

GENERAL CONCLUSIONS ON HORMONES

Steroid hormones have an essential role in the growth, differentiation and function of many tissues in both animals and man. It is established by animal experimentation that modification of the hormonal environment by gonadectomy, by pregnancy or by exogenous administration of steroids can greatly increase or decrease the spontaneous occurrence of tumours or the induction of tumours by applied carcinogenic agents. In man also, there is evidence that differences in endogenous hormone levels may be associated with differences in tumour incidence. It is possible, therefore, that the incidence of human tumours could be increased or decreased by a specific mode of exogenous hormone administration, but this cannot be predicted.

For an administered oestrogen seriously to perturb the hormonal environment of man, the intake must be of the same order as, or greater than, the amounts of oestrogens produced endogenously (Table V). The intake of steroids for effective contraceptive medication has to be sufficient to disturb the hormonal environment, and in fact such a disturbance is a requisite of fertility inhibition. The possibility that a carcinogenic risk may be involved in such medication must therefore be considered. For example, the minimum effective dose of diethylstilboestrol of 6 µg/kg bw/day for mammary carcinogenesis in mice is of the same order as the doses used for therapy in women (0.5-5 mg/day). At the same time, it should be remembered in regard to both oestrogens and progestins in contraceptive medication that the steroid hormones of pregnancy have actions similar to those of the contraceptive agents.

Animal data

Administration of the natural oestrogens, oestradiol-17β and oestrone, increases the incidence of tumours in a number of organs in a variety of animal species. Data on the synthetic oestrogen diethylstilboestrol indicate that this compound has a carcinogenic potential comparable with those of oestradiol-17β and of oestrone, and there is no evidence to suggest that its carcinogenic properties are due to some special biological function other than its oestrogenic activity, which is of the same order as that of oestradiol-17β. The other synthetic oestrogens, ethinyloestradiol and mestranol, have been shown to be carcinogenic in a limited number of animal studies, but there is no reason to suppose that they are more or less carcinogenic than are other oestrogens at comparable levels of oestrogenic activity. Because of lack of experimental data no attempt has been made to show a relationship between carcinogenic potential and oestrogenic activity for any of the compounds considered.

The majority of experimental animal treatments with oestrogens, which have resulted in carcinogenesis, have been at very high dose levels. There is inadequate information at present, however, to indicate the minimum dose requirements, and these could be much lower than those commonly employed in animal studies.

In the case of the natural progestin, progesterone, there is not much evidence that it has a carcinogenic potential _per se_. There is, however, evidence that low doses of progesterone administered over long periods act in combination with carcinogenic agents such as some viruses or chemicals. In part, therefore, the hazard of long-term administration of synthetic progestins is comparable with that associated with progesterone in increasing the incidence of tumours due to other agents. This is dependent on the degree of progestational activity possessed by the compound in question relative to its other hormonal characteristics.

The synthetic progestins, such as norethynodrel and norethisterone, have some carcinogenic potential in animal systems even when administered alone. This is increased by combination with oestrogens. The progesterone analogue, chlormadinone acetate, has not demonstrated carcinogenic properties when given alone to rodents. When combined with oestrogens, its carcinogenic potential appears to parallel that of the oestrogenic component Evidence for its tumour-inducing capacity in the canine breast does not seem to be sufficient evidence, alone, for the prohibition of its use in women (see p. 29).

There is no evidence at present to suggest that steroid hormones are ultimate carcinogens; on the contrary, all the evidence suggests that they act, in part at least, by modification of pituitary hormone secretion in which prolactin is a factor. In general, it appears that steroids increase the probability of tumour occurrence in those tissues normally responsive to stimulation by such steroids.

Human data

Steroid hormones, such as those considered in this monograph, have been and are used extensively in human therapy. When they are used for the treatment of disseminated cancer such as that of the breast, prostate and endometrium, their effect on tumour growth and the severity of side-effects are the major considerations. In the use of steroid therapy for less vital reasons (for example, menstrual disorders, menopausal syndrome, pregnancy maintenance, osteoporosis, protein anabolism, gonadal deficiency), however, the question of carcinogenic hazard becomes more pertinent. With the continuing development of steroid use for the control of conception, the question of possible carcinogenic hazards has become of major importance.

As stated in the general introduction (see p.11), "at the present time no attempt can be made to interpret the animal data directly in terms of human risk since no objective criteria are available to do so". There is, therefore, no substitute for direct observation in the human being, although the animal experimentation provides important clues as to where one should look for human risks. Epidemiological studies to explore the possibility of a carcinogenic effect of administered oestrogens and progestins in man, however, suffer from two major difficulties. Firstly, the interval between the commencement of administration and the possible appearance of cancer is likely to be long. Secondly, to detect a small or moderate change in risk, observations on very large numbers of subjects are required.

With these reservations in mind the following can be said:

1. Diethylstilboestrol

(a) The administration of this drug to women during pregnancy is associated with an increased risk of vaginal or cervical adenocarcinoma in their exposed female offspring.

(b) There may also be an increased risk of endometrial carcinoma in women with gonadal dysgenesis treated with this drug.

(c) It is possible that the administration of the drug therapeutically to men with carcinoma of the prostate increases the risk of cancer of the breast.

2. Other oestrogens

The administration of oestrogens for treatment of the menopausal syndrome and related conditions has not been shown to be associated with a risk of cancer.

3. Oral contraceptives

The administration of these preparations has not as yet been shown to alter the risk of cancer of the breast. The evidence with respect to cancer of the cervix is somewhat less consistent.

CUMULATIVE INDEX TO IARC MONOGRAPHS ON THE EVALUATION
OF CARCINOGENIC RISK OF CHEMICALS TO MAN

Numbers underlined indicate volume and numbers in italics indicate page.

Aflatoxin B1	$\underline{1}$,*145*
Aflatoxin B2	$\underline{1}$,*145*
Aflatoxin G1	$\underline{1}$,*145*
Aflatoxin G2	$\underline{1}$,*145*
Aldrin	$\underline{5}$,*25*
4-Aminobiphenyl	$\underline{1}$,*74*
Aniline	$\underline{4}$,*27*
Aramite^R	$\underline{5}$,*39*
Arsenic	$\underline{2}$,*48*
Arsenic pentoxide	$\underline{2}$,*48*
Arsenic trioxide	$\underline{2}$,*48*
Asbestos	$\underline{2}$,*17*
Auramine	$\underline{1}$,*69*
Benz(c)acridine	$\underline{3}$,*241*
Benz(a)anthracene	$\underline{3}$,*45*
Benzidine	$\underline{1}$,*80*
Benzo(b)fluoranthene	$\underline{3}$,*69*
Benzo(j)fluoranthene	$\underline{3}$,*82*
Benzo(a)pyrene	$\underline{3}$,*91*
Benzo(e)pyrene	$\underline{3}$,*137*
Beryl	$\underline{1}$,*18*
Beryllium	$\underline{1}$,*17*
Beryllium oxide	$\underline{1}$,*17*
Beryllium sulphate	$\underline{1}$,*18*
BHC (technical trades)	$\underline{5}$,*47*
N,N'-Bis(2-chloroethyl)-2-naphthylamine	$\underline{4}$,*119*
Bis(chloromethyl)ether	$\underline{4}$,*231*
1,4-Butanediol dimethanesulphonate	$\underline{4}$,*247*

Cadmium	2,74
Cadmium carbonate	2,74
Cadmium chloride	2,74
Cadmium oxide	2,74
Cadmium sulphate	2,74
Cadmium sulphide	2,74
Calcium arsenate	2,48
Calcium arsenite	2,48
Calcium chromate	2,100
Carbon tetrachloride	1,53
Chlormadinone acetate	6,149
Chlorobenzilate	5,75
Chloroform	1,61
Chloromethyl methyl ether	4,239
Chromic oxide	2,100
Chromium	2,100
Chromium dioxide	2,101
Chromium trioxide	2,101
Chrysene	3,159
Cycasin	1,157
DDD	5,83
DDE	5,83
DDT	5,83
o-Dianisidine	4,41
Dibenz(a,h)acridine	3,247
Dibenz(a,j)acridine	3,254
Dibenz(a,h)anthracene	3,178
7H-Dibenzo(c,g)carbazole	3,260
Dibenzo(h,rst)pentaphene	3,197
Dibenzo(a,e)pyrene	3,201
Dibenzo(a,h)pyrene	3,207
Dibenzo(a,i)pyrene	3,215
Dibenzo(a,l)pyrene	3,224
3,3'-Dichlorobenzidine	4,49

Dieldrin	_5_,125
1,2-Diethylhydrazine	_4_,153
Diethylstilboestrol	_6_,55
Diethyl sulphate	_4_,277
Dihydrosafrole	_1_,170
Dimethisterone	_6_,167
3,3'-Dimethoxybenzidine	_4_,41
3,3'-Dimethylbenzidine	_1_,87
1,1-Dimethylhydrazine	_4_,137
1,2-Dimethylhydrazine	_4_,145
Dimethyl sulphate	_4_,271
Endrin	_5_,157
Ethinyloestradiol	_6_,77
Ethynodiol diacetate	_6_,173
Haematite	_1_,29
Heptachlor	_5_,173
Hydrazine	_4_,127
Indeno(1,2,3-cd)pyrene	_3_,229
Iron-dextran complex	_2_,161
Iron-dextrin complex	_2_,161
Iron oxide	_1_,29
Iron-sorbitol-citric acid complex	_2_,161
Isonicotinic acid hydrazide	_4_,159
Isosafrole	_1_,169
Lead acetate	_1_,40
Lead arsenate	_1_,41
Lead carbonate	_1_,41
Lead chromate	_2_,101
Lead phosphate	_1_,42
Lead subacetate	_1_,40
Lindane	_5_,47
Magenta	_4_,57
Maleic hydrazide	_4_,173
Medroxyprogesterone acetate	_6_,157

Mestranol	6,87
Methoxychlor	5,193
Methylazoxymethanol acetate	1,164
N-Methyl-N,4-dinitrosoaniline	1,141
4,4'-Methylene bis (2-chloroaniline)	4,65
4,4'-Methylene bis (2-methylaniline)	4,73
4,4'-Methylenedianiline	4,79
N-Methyl-N'-nitro-N-nitrosoguanidine	4,183
Mirex	5,203
1-Naphthylamine	4,87
2-Naphthylamine	4,97
Nickel	2,126
Nickel acetate	2,126
Nickel carbonate	2,126
Nickel carbonyl	2,126
Nickelocene	2,126
Nickel oxide	2,126
Nickel subsulphide	2,126
Nickel sulphate	2,127
4-Nitrobiphenyl	4,113
N-{4-(5-Nitro-2-furyl)-2-thiazolyl}acetamide	1,181
N-Nitroso-di-n-butylamine	4,197
N-Nitrosodiethylamine	1,107
N-Nitrosodimethylamine	1,95
Nitrosoethylurea	1,135
Nitrosomethylurea	1,125
N-Nitroso-N-methylurethane	4,211
Norethisterone	6,179
Norethisterone acetate	6,179
Norethynodrel	6,191
Norgestrel	6,201
Oestradiol-17β	6,99
Oestriol	6,117
Oestrone	6,123

Pentachloronitrobenzene	<u>5</u>,211
Potassium arsenate	<u>2</u>,48
Potassium arsenite	<u>2</u>,49
Potassium dichromate	<u>2</u>,101
Progesterone	<u>6</u>,135
1,3-Propane sultone	<u>4</u>,253
β-Propiolactone	<u>4</u>,259
Quintozene	<u>5</u>,211
Saccharated iron oxide	<u>2</u>,161
Safrole	<u>1</u>,169
Sodium arsenate	<u>2</u>,49
Sodium arsenite	<u>2</u>,49
Sodium dichromate	<u>2</u>,102
Sterigmatocystin	<u>1</u>,175
Stilboestrol	<u>6</u>,55
Streptozotocin	<u>4</u>,221
Strobane[R]	<u>5</u>,219
TDE	<u>5</u>,83
Terpene polychlorinates	<u>5</u>,219
Testosterone	<u>6</u>,209
Tetraethyllead	<u>2</u>,150
Tetramethyllead	<u>2</u>,150
o-Tolidine	<u>1</u>,87

www.ingramcontent.com/pod-product-compliance
Ingram Content Group UK Ltd.
Pitfield, Milton Keynes, MK11 3LW, UK
UKHW051259180426
11947UKWH00020B/1796